WRITING BEGINS WITH THE BREATH

WRITING BEGINS

WITH THE

BREATH

Embodying
Your Authentic Voice

LARAINE HERRING

Shambhala
Boston & London
2007

Shambhala Publications, Inc.
Horticultural Hall
300 Massachusetts Avenue
Boston, Massachusetts 02115
www.shambhala.com

14 13 12 11 10 9 8 7 6

Printed in the United States of America

∞ This edition is printed on acid-free paper that meets the
American National Standards Institute z39.48 Standard.
♻ This book is printed on 30% postconsumer recycled paper.
For more information please visit www.shambhala.com.
Distributed in the United States by Penguin Random House LLC
and in Canada by Random House of Canada Ltd

Designed by Graciela Galup

Library of Congress Cataloging-in-Publication Data
Herring, Laraine, 1968–
Writing begins with the breath: embodying your authentic voice /
Laraine Herring.—1st ed.
p. cm.
Includes bibliographical references.
ISBN 978-1-59030-473-0 (alk. paper)
1. Authorship—Psychological aspects. I. Title
PN171.P83H47 2007
808′.02019—dc22
2007012971

For my students and teachers

CONTENTS

PART THREE

EMBRACING WHAT AND
WHERE YOU ARE

ACKNOWLEDGMENTS

In deep gratitude to:

Alma Luz Villanueva, Gayle Brandeis, Jeffrey Hartgraves, Robin Craig, Gus Brett, and Mary Sojourner for heart guidance and ears to listen while I babbled on endlessly about this book.

Gayle Brandeis and Jeffrey Hartgraves for insight and guidance in the earliest drafts, Keith Haynes for invaluable editing assistance, and Cain Carroll for generous feedback on the yoga principles and tone of the book.

Eric Walrabenstein at Yoga Pura in Phoenix, Arizona, and Cain and Revital Carroll at Yoga Shala in Prescott, Arizona, for teaching me not just a new language, but a new way of being in this world.

Soapstone writing retreat for snow, solitude, and stillness.

Yavapai College for space, time, and support.

Linda Roghaar, my agent, for believing in the project and in me, and Jennifer Brown at Shambhala for wisdom, patience, and direction.

My Prescott community: Carolina, Tracy, Ramona, and Grace for Big Love.

Keith, for more than I can ever say.

And always, my students, past and present, for opening their hearts to their writing and their lives. You have been one of the great gifts of my life.

WRITING BEGINS WITH THE BREATH

INTRODUCTION

The Seeker, the Sought, and the Space In-Between

A musician must make music, an artist must paint, a poet must write, if he is to be ultimately at peace with himself. What one can be, one must be.

ABRAHAM MASLOW

IN THE WINTER OF 2003, I was accepted into a three-week solitary writer's residency on the Oregon coast. The brochure said the cabin was "modern," but that the resident should be comfortable with solitude in the wilderness. The cabin had electricity, a stove, a shower. The heat came from the wood-stove, which came with three single-spaced pages of operation instructions. I could follow directions. I didn't anticipate any problems. I had lived in Phoenix since 1981 and was eager for water, cold, and clouds.

I arrived on December 21 to sun and more shades of green than I had ever thought possible. The earth was so damp it sunk down under my boot, the softest carpet I had ever stepped on. The unfamiliar smell of damp, decaying wood and leaves awakened something primal in me. Bugs lived in the tree stumps, and salmon still swam in Soapstone Creek, which ran directly beside the cabin. The rush of the winter water was louder than television static. I had not seen moving fresh water since 1980, just before I moved to Phoenix.

It's hard to explain what living in Phoenix is like. Many people move there for the weather, and while it's true you won't shovel snow off your roof, you will soon find yourself trapped in your air-conditioned house or car eight months out of the year. You will find yourself buying very expensive window treatments to keep the sun out of your house. You'll create your own hibernation den in bright sunlight.

As oppressive as the weather is in Phoenix, one thing it is not is a consideration. Everyone knows it will be sunny and hot, except for the four months when it is sunny and not quite as hot. Weather—the moods of the earth—is not a factor in the lives of Phoenicians.

The third day I was in Oregon, it began to snow along the coast. In those first three days, I had seen more water falling from the sky, rushing under bridges, cresting in the ocean, than I had seen in the previous twenty-four years. Water was amazing. It was every bit as powerful as my beloved fire, yet it had the quiet, patient strength to sculpt rock. Locals told me the snow would stop soon. They told me, "It never snows here!" At first, it was beautiful. I was confident it would indeed stop soon because I had planned several trips to Portland to pay homage to Powell's, the largest used bookstore in the United States.

Snow still fell the day I planned to go to Portland. An unfamiliar quiet hung in the woods. In order to get to Portland, I had to travel through two mountain passes I later learned were known as "snow zones." I didn't think it would be a problem. Portland was only seventy-two miles away, and it *never* snowed in Portland. I decided to go, even though it was snowing, because it was the day I had scheduled to go, and the weather had never before dictated anything to me. I packed my coffee, my cell phone, and my Mapquest directions to Powell's. On the way to the car, I slipped, for the third time in as many days, on the icy steps. My head led the way, until my feet slipped and I fell, again, forced to remember I walked on the earth by the grace of the earth, not by the will of my ego.

The compact rental car was frozen. I stood in front of it, gloved hand awkwardly holding my cup of coffee, as if I could will the ice to melt away from the locks. I had never encountered such a thing. I must have assumed the snow would somehow fall around the rental car so my passage would be clear and easy.

By the time I got into the car and onto the winding highway, the snowfall was heavier. "It never lasts by the coast," the brochure said. I was holding on to that belief, even though I couldn't keep the wipers moving fast enough to see. I reached the turnoff to US-26 after forty-five minutes. The fact that I had managed to travel only seven miles in forty-five minutes did not deter me. No one else was out. This did not deter me either. I turned right, past a one-stop shop that had closed due to the weather, and headed east to Portland, visions of floors of used books dancing in front of my eyes.

The first thing I learned was that in Phoenix, I must have driven with only half of myself present. Roads are always dry, safe, and well maintained. The second thing I learned is that cars take longer to stop on ice than on dry pavement. I knew this intellectually, but until the awareness moved into my body, it didn't really sink in. The snowfall increased. I couldn't see the road anymore. The evergreen trees that lined the highway were heavy with snow of the kind I had only seen in movies. The yellow, diamond-shaped sign with the words "SNOW ZONE" on it was covered with snow, revealing only "S W

NE" to drivers. I kept waiting for the snow to stop simply because I wanted it to.

I witnessed my psyche split and my Ego take over all operational activities. It chattered like a monkey and took on the form of a cartoonish reptile. My Ego was going to Powell's. It chanted the mantra over and over. "Powell's. Book Mecca. Powell's. Book Mecca." It was going whether it killed us both or not. "Powell's. Book Mecca." It salivated. Money to spend. Books to touch. The scent of stories to inhale in the dust of the stacks.

Somewhere, in a calm detached corner of my being, I said, "You are going to crash the car, and we are going to freeze to death in a ravine before help arrives." My Ego responded by following even closer to the car in front of us. The car in front braked. My Ego braked and the car spun. We were facing oncoming traffic. I held my breath. "Turn around and go back," I whispered. But, ever true to its mission, my Ego turned the car back to the east and kept going.

Apparently, I had entered the never-ending snow zone. I looked at my odometer. Four miles. I remembered something my mother said when we would walk along the beach in North Carolina. "Don't use up all your energy on the walk forward. You have to remember to get back." If I turned around now, I'd have to go back through everything I had just crossed. How safe could that possibly be? I began to think of the snow zone as the great birth canal. Treacherous. Wet and slippery. But I would emerge on the other side new and fresh and surrounded by three floors of books. The Universe intended for me to go to Powell's. It had delivered me so far. It would take me to the end.

Another three miles and thirty minutes passed. The awareness began to creep in that I might not make it to Portland that day even if I didn't have an accident. Seventy-two miles at three miles per hour is a lot of hours. I should turn back. The visions of books dancing in my head took on vocal chords—seductive sirens of the printed page. Their energy—a white light of road safety and skid-free stops—would guide me safely to Powell's. I had turned the radio off to better hear the machinations of my Ego, so I didn't hear the news that it was snowing in Portland (which it never does). I didn't know Portland had shut down its public transportation system for the first time in twenty-three years so that befuddled DOT employees could *find* chains for the buses. But even if I had known that, I would still have kept going. I know my Fire.

Then came the elk. He just stood there, frozen like my car had been. My Ego and the elk made eye contact. The elk wasn't moving. So, I thought, it was to be death by elk. I would have laughed if there had been more time. I slammed on the brakes, and the car spun around and around, like swirls of marshmallow in cocoa. I ended up nose out in a snowbank. There was no sign of the elk. My Ego cowered in the backseat, strapped in with both seatbelts. The white light and angelic harmonies of the beckoning books had disappeared. I had a half-tank of gas left. The back wheels spun, unable to find traction in the fresh snow. If I turned off the engine, I would freeze to death. It was twenty-eight degrees. I didn't know how long it would take a Phoenician in one pair of cheap wool socks, a sweatshirt, sweatpants, and four-dollar driving gloves to freeze to death.

My Ego had gone dead silent. I remembered hearing a story on National Public Radio about a woman found in her car in a snowdrift after the spring thaw in North Dakota. She had written on napkins every day she could until she died. She wasn't found for five months. I was not going to die sixty-one miles from Book Mecca. Surely no faithful disciple would be allowed to come so far, only to perish in frozen water. Rock, paper, scissors. Or in this case, earth, water, fire. Guess what. Frozen water kills fire.

It was only fifteen minutes before friendly Oregon folks with four-wheel drive stopped and helped me push out of the drift. I pointed the car west, toward the coast, where surely it was not snowing anymore, and inched back to my cabin where I was certain I would not be able to light the woodstove, but at least I would be able to use the bathroom.

I saw in that failed trip to Powell's how much sheer will I had—how much I thought Earth would alter her weather patterns for me, how much my natural pattern, my habit, was to force forward like a bulldozer, whether it made sense or not. And, I saw how much suffering I incurred simply with my mind. I saw in that day why my novel had stagnated, why I was drowning in a sea of English 101 classes and after-school programs, why I had few intimate relationships. I didn't know how to surrender. I didn't know how to "be." I only knew how to "do," and I knew in that moment that my writing would never breathe on its own if I didn't learn how to let go.

Sitting alone in a snowstorm for the first time in my life, I realized how out of balance I had become in my writing and in my life. In Oregon, I practiced yoga every day in front of the woodstove. I listened to my mind. I stayed with the discomfort and unfamiliarity of snow piling up around the windows. I stayed with the discomfort of knowing that I did not have the skills necessary to venture out into this weather. I stayed with my loss of control to see where it took me, and I arrived back at the writing process.

This book is about stopping long enough to discover your own deep writing practice. Underneath my down comforter, listening to the rush of the full icy creek below the window, I learned that deep, authentic writing does not come from the intellect, as one might expect. Deep writing comes from our bodies, from our breath, and from our ability to remain solid in the places that scare us. It comes from merging with what we are writing—from dissolving our egos so that the real work can emerge through us, without our conditions for success attached to it.

Part of the work of finding your own deep writing comes from awareness of the body. It's easy for us to forget the importance of the body in the writing process. Because words and language are constructs of the mind, we often associate the writing process only with the intellect. Indeed, language does come from the mind, but the stories that spring from the authentic voice that is ours and ours alone come from within own bodies. Our cells have memories. Our bodies have stored all of our experiences—those expressed and unexpressed, even those forgotten. They are there, waiting for us.

When we realize we are carrying these stories with us, expressing them is the next natural step. Some of us carry stories of grief or betrayal. Some of romantic love or hope. Some of us have war stories—in military combat or within our relationships. Some of us have birthing stories, some dying stories. Whatever stories we have, they are organically connected to our physical bodies. Cultivating that connection—that pathway between our heads and our bodies—creates deep writing. Part of what can be frightening about deep writing is that it forces us to dive into those areas of our beings that we have consciously or unconsciously shut ourselves off from. It demands of us to move deeper inside and face what we have not wanted to look at.

As writers, we must learn how to manage our mind, our stories, and our body's emotional triggers. We must learn to be still. When we can create a space of stillness around ourselves, we can begin to access the deeper core of our stories.

We can learn to embody our stories *as we write them.* In order to do that, we have to first be present in our own bodies, and we have to learn to quiet our minds so that the writing works, so that the stories inside of us can be heard.

Observing our breath gives us, as writers, an opportunity to truly embody the writing process in our cells. As we witness our breath and become more conscious of its ebbs and flows, we may come to notice that our writing practice also has natural ebbs and flows. Writing practice has moments of great intensity and moments of almost imperceptible movement. As you become aware that your writing is with you all the time, with each inhale and exhale, you'll be able to let yourself dive into the unknown in-between place where your authentic voice lives.

The chapters in this book offer ways to observe your mind and self in the writing process. One way I ask you to do this is through breath and body exercises—just small, easy things to help move blocks in your writing. Though, of course, none of this work is easy. Deep writing emerges from the space between the inhalation and the exhalation, that space in between the doing and the dreaming, our place of power, of mystery, and of authenticity. I hope to help you find and cultivate that space within yourselves. This book is your invitation to move to the in-between space with me.

About the Book

Please don't feel compelled to move linearly through this book, and please don't feel like you must do all of the exercises. I am hoping you'll return to the book again and again, as *you* change and expand. I am hoping something that doesn't work for you today might hold the key for you tomorrow, and vice versa. Writing, like life, is dynamic, not static.

There's no key that fits every lock, nor one lock for every writer. This book will not provide you with definitive answers; rather, I hope it will help you reframe your questions in such a way that the answers—your answers—become obvious. You don't need any special, expensive tools. You don't need to invest in a laptop or subscribe to a scholarly journal. You do need to show up. It might be helpful for you to have a process journal where you can write down your feelings and responses to some of the exercises and questions. A journal can be very helpful for reflection and giving you an easy place to find your thoughts. Among many things, writing is a way of thinking. Through writing, we discover our thoughts and our ideas. Through writing we can deconstruct and dissolve those same thoughts and ideas. We can gain clarity, focus, and lightness.

I invite you to return to the breath throughout this book. Cultivate a relationship with your breath as you cultivate a deeper relationship with your writing. Returning to the rise and fall of breath, bringing a level of conscious awareness to a predominantly involuntary action, reins in the scattered nature of our thoughts and grounds us in our bodies, squarely in the present moment where we must remain if we are to write deeply.

Begin to pay attention to the energy of breath. When you inhale, you take into your body the flow of energy around you. At the top of the inhale, there is a slight pause where the outer breath merges with the inner breath. When you exhale, you surrender to the world around you, trusting that as you let go you will be filled back up. This trust and surrender is essential to your writing practice. The more you hold, the less you can express authentically. The pause at the end of the exhale allows the outer world to hold the breath, merging into wholeness. In the places of pausing, we simply experience. No striving. No thinking. No judgment. We just experience things as they are. From this place, we live uncontrived moments. From this place, we write authentically. As you allow your breath to naturally rise and fall within your body, practice an awareness of trust that the breath will continue to sustain you. As your natural breath comes forth, your natural voice will begin to find its way to the surface. Nature works without your control. Deep writing does as well.

To help you deepen your practice, I've given you a series of Touchstones at the end of each chapter, as well as some scattered Body Breaks. These exercises are designed specifically to work with the topic of the individual chapters, but I hope you'll find they are much more than that. Many of the prompts can be used for both personal journal work and deep character work. For example, if the prompt is: "To me change means . . . ," you can replace the "me" with the voices of your characters. Don't be afraid to stretch and bend the exercises. They are just springboards for your own deep-sea diving. The Body Breaks will help you stay grounded in your physical form while you're in the process of reading, creating further integration.

This book is not a craft book. It is a process book. Let this book supplement your knowledge of craft, of grammar, of storytelling. This book represents the part of the writing process that lurks underneath the more concrete aspects of style and plot. You can't properly punctuate and shape material that isn't fully formed. Conversely, if you don't shape and punctuate that dynamic, fire-born material, your work won't communicate as it should.

Continue to look for more knowledge both outside yourself and within yourself. Read. Read. Read. And recognize that writing, like all of life, is an exploration. Every tool you pick up has value, but every tool won't work in every situation. Hammers are great for nailing, but not so great for sawing.

Respect your writing enough to gather tools from many different sources, with the final and most important source, yourself. Delight in language—yours and the words of others. Play in the park with your stories and poems, but don't forget to send them to boot camp for structure and focus.

Now, let's begin at the beginning. Beginner's mind. Open mind. Open heart. See the world, your life, and your work with wonder and awe. Breathe deeply into your body, your lungs, your internal organs. The oxygen is giving you fuel. It's bathing the body with energy. What more could you possibly desire?

PART ONE

FOCUSING THE MIND

Asking is the beginning of receiving. Make sure you don't go to the ocean with a teaspoon. At least take a bucket so the kids won't laugh at you.

JIM ROHN

With each inhale, our lungs stretch open, our rib cages swell, our hearts expand. Each inhale is a new beginning, a clean slate. At the start of a writing project, we have this same clean slate. The possibilities for what we can accomplish are truly limitless. Many writers find great delight in the conception stage of their work. But for others, the awareness of their own writing potential can be overwhelming, causing them to freeze, hold their breath, shut down.

Whether the blank page causes you to smile or hide under the covers, part 1 will provide you tools for growth. Here, we'll work with quieting the mind so that you can get the most out of your beginning stages. Inspiration doesn't descend like a lightning bolt from the gods. Inspiration comes instead from a steady breath, a solid foundation, and a commitment to the process. From a grounded breath, freedom blooms. From a grounded breath, your stories and poems can dance themselves awake on the page.

This section also helps you gain awareness of your thoughts. Where thoughts go, energy goes. The more mindful you are of the scattered nature of your thoughts, the more you'll be able to gently refocus yourself as you watch your stories grow. As fast as one thought blows away, another blows in. Release them one by one.

This section gives you the tools to play, explore, laugh, ask questions, and delight in the unexpected. Don't be afraid to start again and again. And most importantly, don't be afraid to surprise yourself.

Body Break

Sit comfortably with your spine straight. Breathe normally for a few breaths. Then, close your right nostril with your right thumb. Inhale fully through your left nostril. Release the right nostril and close the left nostril with the right ring finger. Exhale slowly and fully though the right nostril. Keeping the left nostril closed, inhale fully through the right nostril. Close the right nostril and exhale through the left. This completes one round. Repeat up to eight times. Then relax and breathe normally.

Why? Increases mental clarity, balances the left and right hemispheres of the brain, and evokes a sense of relaxed vitality.

1

RISK

And the day came when the risk it took to remain tightly closed in a bud was more painful than the risk it took to bloom.

ANAÏS NIN

THIS MORNING, a great blue heron lands on the rooftop outside my office window. Its legs are sticks, belly oblong, neck a cobra. It stands on one foot. I see its feathers lifting in the wind, its beak opening and closing. It shifts from foot to foot, then pushes off into the sky. Every moment a risk, a trust, a commitment.

I was first introduced to the concept of risk in writing in graduate school. The memoirist Michael Datcher was giving a seminar where he discussed the psychological fallout from a book. He said that everything you write, if it is authentic, will have fallout, and then he asked us, "What are you willing to risk to tell your stories?" And he implied that if we played it safe, hedged our bets, we were doing a disservice to our art. He wanted us to metaphorically slice ourselves open and see what oozed out. I've never forgotten that lecture, partly because it had never occurred to me that I needed to make myself so vulnerable. It's an obvious concept now, but at that time, I had very little idea what he was actually talking about. In retrospect, I see that this element of *personal risk* is what is missing from virtually all "failed" writing attempts. The writer tries to play it safe, tries to couch what he's doing in layers of deep, and often beautifully phrased crap. The reader spots this right away, though she may not be able to articulate what she's picking up. She only knows she's lost interest. The writing teacher needs to be able to point out—hey, this is a little thick here, don't you think? What if you cut out these first ten, twenty pages and started with this feeling here? The author usually begins formulating resistance to this idea right away. That's OK. The writer, if he is to write, will move through that resistance, find the feeling, and expand upon it.

To nonwriters, personal risk in writing sounds very bizarre. After all, we're not ice climbing or running the Colorado River in a raft made of three planks. We're sitting down and moving our hands. Not so much risk there. But the risk of writing is an internal risk. You brave the depths of your own being and then, oh my, bring it back up for commentary by the world. Not the work of wimps.

Many writers would likely rather climb Mt. Fuji than go *in there*, but *in there* is precisely where you must go. And here's the kicker—you can't really prepare for what's in there because you don't *know* all that's in there. You can research hiking conditions on Mt. Fuji. You can bring proper equipment. You can make sure your body is in appropriate shape. In short, you can plan. But you can't map out the inner world ahead of time; you can only tell us what you experienced after you've been there and returned. Each time you go, you'll find something new. As you explore, reflect, and write on what you're finding, you'll be shown new things. "Oh, I thought I was done with that," doesn't really exist *in there*. There's always a level beneath. Your writing will tell you what you're mining *in there*, but you can't usually see it at the time.

Think of your work, no matter what genre, as a dialogue first with yourself. You don't come out with these dialogues and publish them as is, straight from *in there*. That's for your eyes only. But you can take the belly of what you bring back, craft it, and put it out in the world. The reader will recognize that you've been on the journey, even if she can't identify what the journey is. The reader will know that you risked it all, and she will stick with the story.

Body Break

Take a moment to lie down on your back on the floor. If your back is tender, you can bend your knees and keep the soles of your feet on the floor, or you can put a pillow underneath your knees. Allow your arms to rest beside you, palms up. Close your eyes. You may wish to place an eye pillow over your eyes if you have difficulty keeping them closed. Lie here as long as you like. This is a place of deep relaxation and awareness. You are not asleep, but you are still.

Why? This posture helps stimulate the imagination. Also, because you're on your back, your heart is open, allowing you to experience both vulnerability and surrender. Your body is experiencing a place of safe openness—a place of trust from which you can dare to risk.

I often write on student papers, "What is at stake for your protagonist? Why here? Why now?" These are important characterization questions to consider. What is the urgency of that story? Why is it imperative that you begin the story in that place and time, rather than in the following day or in a neighboring city? If you find that you could enter your story dream at any random spot, then likely you have focus issues to think about. We choose the point of entry into our stories based on the impact we want to create for the reader. There is only one point of entry for every story. To change that point of entry changes the story.

These questions also apply to the writer. Why here? Why now? What is the urgency in this story for me? What do I want to learn, uncover, discover, about my life or myself? Some stories have more obvious answers to these questions than others. But what of the novelist who has a persistent pull toward tulips, or who hears the whisperings of an old man in her ear? Does she know what she's risking? Likely not at the beginning, but the risk will become evident through the writing. If there is nothing at stake for the author, there won't be enough energy to sustain a longer project. Novels have a defining question that gets resolved at the end. If the writer knows all the answers along the way, there is no joy of the discovery.

There are levels of risk. A person who has never shared work out loud before is taking a huge risk simply by offering up her words. But a writer who has been writing for many years, producing and sharing, must continue to go down deep in her heart and keep excavating the things that haunt her. She must continue to challenge herself so her work will challenge others. Writing is both an act of power and surrender. Passion and discovery. It is a tug at your soul that continues to pull you forward, even as you go kicking and screaming.

When you discover what you're risking, you may "block." Understand that it is not the writing itself that is blocked. The term "writer's block" shifts the responsibility away from the author onto the writing. The writing is not blocking you. You are blocking the writing. This is a very empowering reframing. If you're doing the blocking, then you can do the unblocking.

No more waiting on the great god of writing to release the faucet of inspiration. How liberating!

The first step when you find yourself stuck is to become aware of what is being blocked. What point have you reached in your work? What is the next scene, next poem, next essay? Can you identify some piece of the next step that contains something you might not be ready or willing to address yet? Writing has a sneaky way of pushing us out of our comfort zone. When we "let it loose," like a Bengal tiger, it goes right for the raw meat. We set up our defenses and then hope for a quick diversion from the center of our stories. But we can't continue to do that and still be in service to our projects. Our work deserves our full attention, our presence, and our commitment.

I've noticed that the closer I get to the heart of the story, the quicker and more solid the "block" seems to feel. Over time, I've observed this pattern in myself, and so I recognize it for what it is: a fear-based pattern. I don't want to sit in my chair and write these stories because they affect the way I am feeling, so I won't. That's the block. And I can do something about that. There is no secret code to breaking through the blocks, but there is one surefire way, and it's the way no one really wants to use, but it works. Write. Stay with the discomfort. Stay with the uncertainty. Stay with the emotions that a scene or a memory might conjure up for you. Stay with the work. It'll guide you back home.

Touchstones

1. Journal for at least fifteen minutes on each of the following prompts:
   - When I am at a crossroads, I . . .
   - Change means . . .

· Fear means . . .
· Risk means . . .

2. Strong writing is concrete writing. Look back over your four journal responses and identify the abstract idea in each one. Then create a concrete image for that abstraction. Using a fresh piece of paper, begin a new creative piece starting with one or more of the concrete images you've come up with. For example, if one of your abstract ideas for "change" is "it's scary," take "it's scary" and find a concrete image for it, such as "the crawlspace smelled of skunk and ashes." Begin a new piece with the specific image and see where it takes you.

3. Freewrite a list of fears and/or reasons why you are not always truthful in your writing. If all of those reasons came to pass, what would happen?

2

AUTHENTICITY

I will not stick one word next to the other like graves as all the dead poets did. I want to see the words floating in the white lake of the page like scattered ashes.

M. V. MINER

WHAT DOES IT MEAN TO WRITE and live authentically? I think there are many parts to authentic living and writing, but the crux of them both is the ability to stand in your own body. I know that might sound ridiculous. If you're not standing in your own body, then whose body are you standing in? Simply standing up and standing *in* are not the same thing. Let's try it.

Stand in a solid position. First, press your feet firmly into the floor. Lift your toes and fan them out, letting them settle into the floor. Allow your weight to equally distribute among the four corners of both feet. Keep your knees soft and un-locked. Feel your feet and knees in line with your hip bones, feet pointing straight forward, parallel to each other. Activate your inner thigh muscles and allow your tailbone to glide toward the floor. This will release your lower back. Lift your shoulders up and then let them settle back down. Relax, soften the jaw, and breathe slowly and deeply. In yoga, this is called mountain pose.

Now, simply stand there. What do you feel? You may feel awkward at first. We spend a lot of time standing with more weight on one foot than the other. We spend a lot of time slouched. We spend a lot of time sucking in our bellies so we appear thinner. What do you notice in your own body? Mountain pose is a simple practice you can do anywhere. Standing in line at the grocery store. Fueling your vehicle. Making a presentation at the office. The more you are able to become aware of how you stand, the more other things will become apparent to you. Things like, wow, I'm not standing straight. I'm leaning more toward my right side or my left side. My lower back hurts. My shoulders are always up around my ears rather than relaxed down my back. My feet are always at an angle, not pointed straight ahead.

What value is there in knowing these things? Awareness. We must begin to make the connection between the authentic self and the physical form. Often, writers tend to live in their heads, with their bodies as convenient vehicles for transporting those heads. If we spend all our time in our heads, not only do we have to deal with all those messy thoughts spinning around, but we'll soon find ourselves seeking solutions to all our problems and navigating our lives through only one vehicle: the mind. The mind is not meant for all that work. The mind is a gigantic data processor and can only work with the data it has in it, so creative solutions must come from outside the mind.

We experience shifts in perceptions through our skin. We *feel* a new awareness, and then we can store it in our minds for future reference. It simply doesn't work the other way around. We can't think it before we feel it. Many writers talk about getting new ideas or solving plot problems while on a walk, or in the shower, or in their dreams. When they are not focusing the machine of the mind on the problem, answers can surface through other channels. Deep writing requires you to access all your channels, not just one.

Standing in your own body helps open the throat for the opportunity to speak with your own voice. It also helps to move you out of your thinking center and into a place of feeling and sensation. It's in the place of feeling that you are present. Thoughts keep you in the past or the future. We can think about a mountain as a metaphor for writing as well. A mountain is solid, stable, present. It is a foundation of earth for life of all kinds. The foundation of your writing is your practice, your consistent showing up to the page, your awareness of your relationship with your words and language. The stronger that foundation, the more forms of life it can sustain.

We have been well-schooled not to write authentically. We have been taught to write what we think teachers want to read. We have been taught to speak what we think people in authority want to hear. We have been taught to mimic, to parrot, and we have seen those who write or speak outside the established rubrics suffer the consequences. We have also been taught, in myriad ways, to hide our authentic voice because we are afraid (and often rightly so) of being too vulnerable. We are afraid of being exposed for (fill in the blank). We are afraid that if we're writing a novel, our mother/father/daughter will think *we* are that main character who is doing those despicable things. And so we self-censor and ultimately sabotage our work.

How do you know when you are, well, *you*? The most obvious answer is the most vague—you know when you know. But *how* do you know? You practice your writing. You allow yourself to move deeper and deeper into the heart of your pieces. You stand beside yourself, detached yet present, as you journey deep inside. You test yourself, as you bring forth poem after poem and story after story from within you. You honestly assess your work. Ask yourself these questions:

> Is this the truth? (Not literal truth, but the truth
>   of that work).
> What have I left out?
> Why have I left that out?
> What would happen if I added that which I left
>   out back in?
> Where have I written *around* the story?
> What is the question of the story?
> Have I addressed the question of the story, or
>   have I avoided it?

You'll begin to see your own patterns. You'll not only see a pattern in the larger questions of your work, but you'll see a pattern in the way you avoid an issue. You'll notice if you tie up the ending too fast. You'll notice if you skip over the most important (and risky) scenes of the book in favor of quick exposition. You'll notice if your characters are continually in the same places of stuck-ness. Don't judge what you notice. Just notice. This line of deeper questioning will lead you to your authentic voice.

I've had students tell me they didn't want to read because they were afraid they'd "steal" something they read. It's really not possible outside of direct plagiarism. There are hundreds of thousands of boy meets girl stories out there. Each author tells that story in his or her own way. It can't be any different than that. You, as a novice writer, are seeking the voice that is yours and yours alone. In the beginning, there is often imitation. Read a lot of Anaïs Nin and find yourself writing long diary entries. Read a lot of Hemingway and find yourself writing in a short, clipped style. That is OK. You are learning. You cannot be Nin or Hemingway. You can only be you. And that "you" can be found underneath the din of competing voices (teachers, partners, friends, coworkers, other authors). You're in there. Most of us are just out of practice listening.

Stand in your body. Speak with your voice. At first, you may feel awkward standing properly, completely on the earth. At first, you may only be able to croak out a few words or phrases through the pen or through your throat that are authentically you. You may find yourself struggling for a focus, struggling for your voice. This is an essential part of the writer's growth process. You're not born the next Toni Morrison. You cultivate your voice over the course of your life, just like you cultivate the other aspects of a balanced life. You learn what you most need to say as you engage in a deeper relationship with yourself, which is the source of all your creativity.

Body Break

Tilt your head back slowly. Let yourself settle into this small stretch and opening. Feel what is happening in the throat as you stretch upward. Just notice and feel.

Why? This is a vulnerable position. It is a position of surrender and trust.

Many of us have blocked off the energy flow at our throats. We've learned to stuff our feelings deep inside us. We've learned it's not always safe to speak the truth. We've learned to censor our ideas. Now that you've accepted the challenge of writing, one of your first tasks is to open up this energy center. One of your first tasks is to trust yourself enough to risk it all to access your voice. Be patient with yourself. This is a very sacred time. You are beginning to cultivate an authentic relationship with yourself. You and your writing deserve nothing less.

Touchstones

1. Let's begin with the body. You can do this sitting or standing. If you're sitting down, make sure both feet are pressed firmly into the floor, grounding you. On an inhale, slowly tilt your head back. Don't try to force it back further than it wants to go. Just enjoy a gentle stretch. Continue to breathe slowly and deeply. Notice what you are feeling. Your neck and throat are exposed. This is a vulnerable, heart-opening position. When you are ready, on an exhaling breath, bring your head back to center. Experiment with this as much as you like, taking care not to force movement in your neck. When you are finished, pick up your pen and freewrite for fifteen minutes.

2. Answer this question in your journals: When I sit down to write, what am I trying to do? Now, reverse it: When I sit down to write, what is the writing trying to do?

3. Freewrite on this prompt: If I really listened to my inner voice, I would . . .

4. If everything were stripped away from you—your body, your health, your relationships, your possessions—and you were left with just your authentic face, what experience, lesson learned, or other truth about your only unique singular precious life, would you like to express? Then, try and find an image or two that communicates that idea. Follow the trail of that image and see what you uncover.

5. Freewrite on this prompt: What is most stuck inside me is . . .

3

HUMILITY

Humility is the solid foundation of all the Virtues.

CONFUCIUS

MAYBE YOU REMEMBER the Mac Davis song from the sixties, "Oh Lord It's Hard to Be Humble." The narrator of the song goes on to proclaim his perfection and the unworthiness of others to be around him. True to convention, the narrator gets his comeuppance at the end of the song when the beautiful woman he'd been rating turns around and rates him. It's a typical story of arrogance resulting in a fall. Someone gets "too big for his britches" and has to be taken down a peg, resulting in being humbled. Doesn't sound like a whole lot of fun, does it? In the Western mind, humility seems connected to punishment, but that could hardly be further from the truth. It doesn't help that our word "humiliation" is so close to the word "humility" either.

Humility is a state of questioning. Through humility, through stepping away from yourself enough to allow for surprises and discoveries, you gain understanding of yourself and of others. If you possess humility, it doesn't mean you've somehow gotten in trouble along the way. You are simply in a place of openness and receptivity. You don't know and don't pretend to know what is going to happen next.

Humility helps us in both stages of the writing process. In the prewriting phase, humility gives us unlimited access to the directions our work can go. We aren't holding tight to desire. We approach each component of our work with the detached, open perspective of a child.

> Wow! What could that be? Let's explore it further.
> Who are you?
> Why are you in my story?

We can follow these questions without anxiety because we aren't attached to where they may take us. We're not holding on to thoughts like: "I can't follow this new character because I'm sure my main character is supposed to be Joe." Or, "I can't stop and write about playing a trombone because there's no musical element to my piece." Humility lets us explore openly. It unlocks a wide door into your unconscious. It lets you approach your work with the innocence of a child, still amazed by the caterpillar crawling on the fence. From that place comes deep writing.

I spent several years studying writing as a healing tool during times of grief and loss, and as I was preparing my final thesis, I worked as an intern at a counseling facility. I was fortunate to work with many extraordinary individuals who shared their stories with me. One man in particular stands out. He was in his early eighties and had been married for fifty-three years. His wife had just died and he was having trouble, as one would expect, adjusting to the loss. He came to see me and he brought three huge scrapbooks with him. He wanted to introduce me to his wife. I saw pictures and letters they'd written to each other about the changes in their relationship over the decades. They wrote openly to each other about sex, the possibility of divorce, an affair, a regret, the children, and her illness. Through them all they wrote of love. He told me about the first time he saw her (the parking lot of a grocery store) and how he left a book of Whitman's verse in her car with his name in it. He talked about their routines together as they grew older. The walks around the neighborhood. Gardening. Reading the newspaper. "I miss her touch," he said, then cried. Part of his healing path was to bring his wife and their relationship to life for others. It was essential for him to share these stories with me, to hear an acknowledgment of the relationship and the love, and, in some way, to share the burden of his loss with another person.

Before this man came to my office, I hadn't ever seen a relationship like that. I hadn't believed that a man could love a woman so completely. My own experience at the time had been limited. He showed me that what I *thought* I knew, I didn't know at all. He showed me a new way of seeing—and he gave me the gift of humility. I sank into his stories. I, too, fell in love with his wife as he did all over again. I fell in love with him, and on the last day he came to see me, he gave me a bookmark with a handwritten note on the back: *Believe in what you don't yet understand.* I've returned to those words many times since then, each time taking a different meaning from them.

I share this with you now because I think it illustrates humility. In order to be of service to this man, I had to release what I thought I knew about loss, about relationships, and about the elderly. And because I was so surprised by what he brought to our sessions, I had no choice but to step back and just experience what he had to say. I could hear him because I didn't know what he was going to say next. I don't know if he was helped at all by coming to see me, but he profoundly altered my perspective.

There are no permanent roles. Students can be teachers; teachers can be students—as long as you're open to the possibility.

Touchstones

1. Let's begin with the body once again. This time, we're going to do the opposite of what we did in the previous chapter. You can do this sitting or standing. If you are sitting, make sure both your feet are firmly on the floor, grounding you. Take a few breaths, and when you're ready, on an inhale, slowly allow your chin to move toward your collarbone. Take your time. Head bowing is a traditional posture of humility. Notice the elongation in the back of the neck. Continue to breathe and relax deeper into the stretch. Take care not to force any movements. You might take your hand and touch the back of your neck softly, feeling the vulnerability of the pose. When you're ready, on an exhale, bring your head back to center. Do this a few more times if you like. Then, pick up your pen and freewrite for at least fifteen minutes.

2. Remember a time when you felt amazement. Describe it in detail.

3. What do you believe is impossible? Write a scene or poem in which the impossible becomes possible.

4. What did you used to think was impossible, but has now become possible? Write a scene or poem about that moment of shifting perspectives.

4

CURIOSITY

All explorers are seeking something they have lost. It is seldom that they find it, and more seldom that the attainment brings them greater happiness than the quest.

ARTHUR C. CLARKE

WHAT DOES IT MEAN to be curious? What is the difference between open inquiry and simple nosiness? Why is Curious George rewarded but a curious cat gets killed? Maybe you heard, "You're asking too many questions" when you were growing up; a line that could easily become code for, "Shut up. You're being a pest."

The "Why is the sky blue?" questioning that occurs in childhood never really goes away for the serious writer. More than why is the sky blue, we want to know why Sam can't get along with his mother, why the wounds between the north and south are still bubbling, why Betty is still longing for a man she saw only once at a bus terminal in Saginaw in 1963. These are story-making questions. We follow the trail of "whys" and they unravel the "hows" of our plots. Underneath the surface questions we ask about our characters must lie a persistent seeking. Literature lets us explore and imagine worlds and ideas we might never have been exposed to. Each exposure to unfamiliar lives opens us up. Our minds and our hearts expand when we experience new things, as does each novel or poem we let into our lives.

It's been said that we write to make meaning out of chaos. Through our stories we come to find the patterns in a random universe and from those patterns we find comfort. All writing poses questions. Novels carry many questions. A poem may only carry one, but it could carry many more. Length is not indicative of depth. Often, a writer organizes his work based on the exploration of these questions. And this part is key: the writer cannot approach his work with the answers to the questions firmly in his mind. There is no humility there, no openness, no softness.

The poet and translator Peter Levitt calls this approach a "closed fist." If you already know where you're going, then your mind stops you from letting in possibilities from outside the box and focuses on its predetermined destination. You will, in all likelihood, get to your destination, but the journey won't have been enriched by detours and unexpected synchronicities. If you have already decided what your answers are, you destroy the spark of curiosity that sustains the work. The writing itself becomes drudgery when you are merely moving from point A to point B in the manner you predicted. And if *you're* not curious, the reader won't be curious, which means your book gets put down in favor of the TV. It's *your* curiosity and *your* questioning that first carries the work. It is this stage where the heart begins to beat.

One of my favorite books growing up was *Harriet the Spy*. I fell in love with Harriet and her stacks of notebooks. Her unrelenting commitment to her notebooks and her endless curiosity helped shape my young writer's persona. She wanted to be Mata Hari. I was a little afraid of being captured and tortured, but still I peered in my neighbors' windows, not with malice, but with curiosity. How do they live? Where do they put the sofa? What colors are on their walls? I read the backs of other people's postcards (after all, anything too private would never be put on a postcard, right?). I took notes on my mother, my father, my sister, my cat. I took notes on the changing leaves and the mean boy on the bus and the men of the neighborhood sitting in green-and-white cloth lawn chairs talking about men things as lightning bugs flickered like the cherries on their cigarettes.

One of the most valuable things *Harriet the Spy* gave to me was an early interest in and awareness of the value of reflection. Harriet took sharp, clipped, journalist-style notes on everything. But she also reflected on them. There would be a note, then a reflection. A note; a reflection. It was my first writing class. *What does what I wrote mean? How does it fit? How does it change me?* Go ahead and peek. We're all human with earwax and toe lint. Isn't that much easier than thinking we're all perfect? Go ahead and peek. Really. It's fun.

Part of your job in the prewriting phase is to maintain a consistent curiosity about your work. Where will it go? Where could it go? If I listen to my main character, where will she take me? What if my main character isn't my main character after all? What sort of possibilities does that open up? One question leads organically to the next one. Each one pulls you a layer deeper. A layer closer to the heart of what you have to say.

If you read an author's body of work, you'll be able to easily identify at least three or four, likely more, questions that author worked with for a lifetime. You'll see that it's not about solving for x as much as it's about identifying what x is, why it's there, and whether it is necessary at all. In the prewriting stage you're uncovering/discovering the defining questions of your work. Keep searching for the questions that will open you, stretch you, and pull you out of your comfort zone where you knew all the answers. As you're pulled out of your comfort zone by the threads of curiosity, don't be deterred. Let the writing shock you and undo you. It will ultimately find you and reveal yourself to you.

Your stories will reveal their questions to you when you maintain curiosity and persistence enough to listen. I've looked back at my own work years later and said, wow, that's what I was working with back then! But I wasn't conscious of

---

Body Break

This exercise will focus on the eyes. Sit or stand comfortably. If you wear glasses, remove them. Practice this activity without moving your head. Hold each direction three seconds. In between each direction, close your eyes and rest a moment. Let's begin.

Look up. Look down. Look left. Look right. Look upper left. Look lower right. Look upper right. Look lower left. Reverse the rotation.

Why? This helps strengthen the optic nerves and muscles and helps relieve eye fatigue. Also, by bringing awareness to your eyes, you will help integrate the body with the eye movement. Energy follows intention, so if our eye movements are scattered and unfocused, our thoughts and energy will follow in turn. Cultivate conscious curiosity by enhancing the relationship between your thoughts (your seeking) and your energy. You will also notice that as you consciously change focus by looking up or to the right or left, you will practice letting go of what you just saw and integrating with what is currently in your line of vision.

it then. It's OK not to know, and I think important not to know, all the levels your work is speaking on. Trust it. Show up for it. Like your breath affects far more than your nostrils, your showing up for the writing feeds much more than an outline or initial idea. It wants to be more than you can imagine. Release the golden handcuffs of your ego. It won't serve you here.

I used to have a plush Eeyore cell phone cover. When I taught a class in magical realism, I brought the Eeyore one day. I took out the cell phone and held up the Eeyore and asked the class what they saw. The most obvious answer of course is, "Eeyore." I kept shaking my head. What else do you see? I held the Eeyore in my hand, arm stretched away from my body. People began to think metaphorically and abstractly.

"Childhood."

"Sadness."

"Happiness."

"Simplicity."

I kept shaking my head. What else? What else?

Finally, someone would say, "I see your arm."

Ah.

"Your fingers."

"You."

"The whiteboard."

"The window."

Yes! Yes!

There are times when we must focus, hone in on an object and hang out there. But in the beginning, when you are simply curious, don't limit yourself to what you think the answer might be. We are so trained to identify, classify, and categorize. We solve for x. There are only four possible answers: a, b, c, or d. This approach limits your thinking. The writer must resist the labeling, the quantifying, and the objectifying. When we think we get *the* answer, we stop thinking about the question. But, if we are aware that there is not a single answer, and that we are searching for what is underneath the obvious, we'll keep an open curiosity about ourselves. If we always focus too directly on a single point, we can't see what's around it, no matter how loudly it might be shouting. In this place of seeking, see not just the mountain, but the worms living in the belly of the mountain and the fires that caused the mountain to push up from the sea. Then, see the interconnectedness of the tree roots underneath the soil. All of these things make "mountain," not just the altitude and temperature statistics. And remember this: the question you most want to avoid is the place you need to begin. Onward! (Take your notebook!)

Touchstones

1. What are you curious about? What have you learned through experience, and what have you learned from books? Notice the difference between heart/body learning and head/mind learning.

2. What is your character seeking? Respond with a monologue.

3. Design a treasure hunt for your characters. Start with an object that has significant meaning to the character. Allow the character to focus on that object, describing it, holding it, imagining where it came from or how it came to be in her possession. Then, follow the object where it leads. Let the object, say, a socket wrench, spring you forward to a Rand McNally map of Nebraska. Let the map bounce you into a laundry room off a two-lane road in the Rockies. Keep going. Let object spring to object. Be specific in your descriptions. Enjoy the process. Let curiosity be your guide.

4. Go on your own treasure hunt. Take a walk and jot down things that you're curious about. Do you know the names of all the plants along the way? Do you want to know? What about the building at the corner that seems to house only cats?

5

EMPATHY

When you plant lettuce, if it does not grow well, you don't blame the lettuce. You look for reasons it is not doing well. It may need fertilizer, or more water, or less sun. You never blame the lettuce. Yet, if we have problems with our friends or family, we blame the other person. But if we know how to take care of them, they will grow well, like the lettuce. Blaming has no positive effect at all, nor does trying to persuade using reason and argument. That is my experience. No blame, no reasoning, no argument, just understanding. If you understand, and you show that you understand, you can love, and the situation will change.

THICH NHAT HANH

WALK A MILE IN ANOTHER PERSON'S SHOES and you'll never be the same. As a way of addressing empathy, this adage has been tossed around in various forms for millennia. Since we obviously can only walk in our own shoes, it's easy to see the struggle humans have with empathy. Empathy requires imagination. I feel my flat feet, my aching shoulder, my nearsighted eyes. I can *know about* your sciatica or your allergies to juniper, but I can't experience them firsthand. The task of the writer is to allow the reader to experience fully the lives of people other than themselves. It's impossible, really. But we can come pretty darn close.

A writer without empathy is cold, detached, and preachy. A writer without empathy doesn't explore the unanswerable questions, but rather sticks firmly to what is known, or what she thinks is known. A writer without empathy creates stick-figure characters who represent ideas or judgments rather than people. A writer without empathy cannot create a world where you, the reader, can understand the characters, even if you don't agree with their actions.

This connection is made when the reader recognizes a piece of himself in the characters he is reading about. If a writer only sees herself as good and noble and right, without recognizing that there are things about herself she does not know, and without an awareness that much she thinks she is incapable of she would do in a heartbeat given the right context, she will not be able to find that place of understanding with others' choices. If I am "good" and my villain is "bad," then how can I possibly see a piece of me in him? And if I, as the *author,* can't find a part of myself in that character, then the reader certainly won't.

Empathy is the cornerstone for many of the seemingly innocent craft components. Empathy resides in the heart. We can often intellectually understand the motivations behind someone's actions, but we still carry grudges and judgments against them. When we are able to soften our angles, relax our tensed jaws and tight shoulders, and let the analysis melt into feelings, we have found empathy with that person.

Sculptor John M. Soderberg says,

One of the most crucial human qualities, I believe, is empathy. Given empathy, brutality becomes impossible. Empathy is at the heart of our humanity, and in fact is the heart of our humanity, for it reduces the barriers of race, religion, and creed to items of mild interest, while unlocking our true, inherent human dignity. The act of encapsulating empathy in some medium, be it dance or music, painting or sculpture, simple stories or more complex forms, is my definition of art. The feeling and then the sharing of an emotion or idea—which is the essence of art—is what makes us human.

We share stories not to cause separation, but to create connections. We say, "Hey, this is my world. Does it gel with yours? Do you understand me? How can I understand you?" And so goes the exploration. When you write, you contribute your voice to the international dialogue of the human condition. When you write, you join other voices that are reaching out to one another and to the world. If you shout *at* someone, you'll create distance between you. If you speak *with* that person, there is a chance of creating real connection and as such, effecting real change.

The first step to cultivating empathy with those around us is to cultivate it within ourselves, for ourselves. If we can't extend ourselves compassion, we can't extend it to others. And, if we don't start the journey of knowing ourselves—all of ourselves, not just the parts we feel safe showing the world—then our compassion practice is conditional, based on appropriate behavior. As you begin to accept the shadow inside of you, you can accept the shadow in others. Acceptance doesn't mean condoning actions. It means recognizing that piece of each of us that is purely a human animal, not dressed up to go to church all the time. Can we love that part of us too?

When building characters, one of the first things to work with is motivation. The "why" of things. What made him plant twelve rosebushes in a circle in his backyard? What made her leave her job on the day she was supposed to make partner? We have to consider the reasons behind our characters' actions, and we have to recognize that those reasons often will not jive with our own way of viewing the world. If we can't find a way to empathize with them, we'll judge them, and it's very clear to a reader when an author judges her characters. Judging creates *distance*. Empathy creates connection. Empathy helps us move from an "us and them" mind-set to a "we" mind-set. If stories narrowly reflect our biases and little else, fiction becomes propaganda, and we rob readers of the right and joy to form their own opinions about the characters we present.

Empathy, like forgiveness, doesn't mean that it's OK for people to murder one another. It means we can find our way past the deeds to the human being, and we can discover the basic need that person was trying to meet. We have to be able to understand the need; we don't have to understand or agree with the methodology used to meet the need. After basic human needs of food, air, water, and shelter are met, most of our actions and behaviors stem from a need for love, compassion, touch, understanding, and emotional safety. And remember, love of self is necessary before authentic love for others can occur. So, maybe your character is unable to love himself for whatever reasons you make up for him. Since he can't do that, he can't have a successful relationship with his spouse. He projects his anger at himself onto her and a series of terrible events ensues. If you keep digging, you'll find that

Body Break

CHILD'S POSE OR EXTENDED CHILD'S POSE

Kneel on the floor. Touch your big toes together and sit back on your heels, then separate your knees about as wide as your hips. If you like, you can roll a blanket up and place it between the backs of your thighs and calves, resting your weight on the blanket for a more comfortable position. Exhale and lean forward until your torso rests between your thighs. Feel your sacrum broaden across the back of your pelvis. Lengthen your tailbone away from the back of your pelvis while you lift the base of your skull away from the back of your neck. Lay your arms on the floor alongside your torso with your palms facing up and release your shoulders toward the floor, feeling their weight pull the shoulder blades wide across your back. If this is challenging for your shoulders, you can stretch your arms out in front of you instead, drawing the shoulder blades down the back. Without lifting your hands, place your buttocks back on the heels. Breathe deeply into the back of your torso, feeling the rise and fall of each breath massaging your entire back. Remain in the pose for one to three minutes.

To come up, first lengthen the front torso and then inhale and lift from the tailbone, feeling it press down and into the pelvis.

Why? The pose stretches your hips, thighs, and ankles, and breathing fully into the back of the torso creates an expansion of your awareness of your chest area. Because this is a resting pose, it relieves stress and fatigue and helps your mind to settle down, allowing for greater intimacy and compassion with your truest self.

Caution: Please don't do this pose if you have diarrhea, are pregnant, or have a knee injury.

though the actions and reactions the character engages in are less than compassionate, the heart of the behavior comes from seeking that compassion. We can all relate to that seeking.

We begin by stripping away the outside manifestations of inward desires. Find the innermost cry of the soul. Touch it. Cradle it like a child and welcome it. Do this for yourself as well as for your characters. Go to your bleeding, wounded heart of hearts and instead of saying, as Kurtz does in *Heart of Darkness,* "The horror! The horror!" say, "I welcome you!" All that you see inside you, all that you are—welcome it fully. When we fight something within us (and outside of us), we give it strength. When we embrace it, we dissolve its energy and it no longer has the power over us it had when we "hated" it. Give it a try. Empathy creates connection; judgment creates distance. Choose connection.

When I was in graduate school, we had quite a few seminars titled with some variation of "writing from the other." These were forums and discussions on the appropriateness (or possibility of) writing effectively from points of view different from our own. As you might imagine, any fiction is written from a point of view different from your own, or else it's memoir, and even memoir requires the memoirist to turn himself into a character.

I think it's possible to write from the point of view of any character, any gender, any socioeconomic class. However, you can't do this if you don't recognize that you are a product of your own mythologies, your own gender, and your own socioeconomic class. If I, as a white woman, want to write from the point of view of a black woman, I can't just say, "Oh, she's me, only black." I have to recognize that first, even if I wrote from a white woman's perspective, she wouldn't be "me," and second, I have to move deeper than the racial or gender lines and find the essence of this woman—the humanness of her. Then, I move back up to context. Be respectful. Do your research. Don't make caricatures of religions or regions or races. Don't use your characters to preach. But feel free to travel where your work is taking you.

Imagine a world of writers writing from a place of deep empathy and compassion. What a revolution in literature and in the world! What an opportunity to bring about greater harmony in the world rather than contribute to the conflicts all around us. Work the conflicts out on the page and present an experience for the reader that allows him to think, expand, laugh, and cry. Literature changes lives. Start with yours.

My second novel, *Bone Dance,* went through many incarnations, as all novels do. One of the areas I was struggling with was finding the right point of view for the story. I tried omniscient. I tried third limited. I hung around in first person for awhile, but I was afraid of it, because one of the narrators was male and I wasn't sure how to write a "Guy." I was convinced that Guys were so different from Gals that there was no way I could bridge the gap. I'd be better off writing from a seven-year-old rural Chinese girl's perspective than a Guy's. Ugh.

My friend, the author Mary Sojourner, told me to try writing a sex scene from the first-person point of view of a male who truly loves the companion he is with. Ugh. So, I had to think, "How does a man make love?" And I struggled and I struggled until the obvious answer popped out from behind its curtain. Hey, dummy, men are people too. Wow. I realize this sounds incredibly ridiculous, but I was so wrapped up in the idea that men are different from women that I could no longer see the part of both men and women that was *human* and without gender. Once I got that, the piece fell into place for me, and the novel opened up. I thought about what I, as a woman, notice with a lover. I stayed specific, small, and focused, and voila, I had a Guy, only he was no longer a capital-*G* guy encapsulating all that is masculine (or more accurately, what I believed to be masculine); he was just a guy, a specific guy to me and my story, with his own specific desires, neuroses, patterns. This is a piece of that exercise.

> He thinks of the last time he made love to her, how her mouth had opened right before he slid his tongue inside it, and how he knew then that she was leaving. He thought that he could bite her, hold her head so tightly she would see how much a part of him she was and stay, but he didn't. Instead, he tasted her teeth, her neck, behind her right ear, and held these things in his body. She didn't know he took these things. He caught her hair in his mouth, the sweet sweet taste of girl-shampoo foreign on his tongue, and he held that too.

Simply letting in the idea that a man could truly love a woman opened up my writing and my life. You'll have different blocks than I do, based on your personal experiences and life choices. But we've all got blocks. Choose connection and the distance will dissolve, and you'll be able to laugh at your own beautiful, imperfectly perfect human self.

Touchstones

1. Write a scene from the opposite gender's point of view in which your character makes love to someone he or she has genuine love for. Remember, no one has to see it!

2. Make a list of pivotal moments of change for you. Select one from your list and write in depth about it. If you like, personify the emotions you're working with. Try writing a

dialogue with the emotion/entity/situation that changed you.

3. Personify an inanimate object and an animal. Write a monologue from the point of view of each of the characters. Give them voices, likes/dislikes, desires, just as if they were human. Play!

4. What clans or groups do you recognize? What groups would be difficult for you to be in a room with? Write a dialogue between you and someone from the "opposite" clan. Write it twice—once from your point of view and once from the other person's point of view. Use first person. Try to embody the *person* from the other clan. Try to see the world as *she* sees it, not as you are recording it.

6

ACCEPTANCE

For after all, the best thing one can do when it is raining is let it rain.

HENRY WADSWORTH LONGFELLOW

REMEMBER THE OLD COUNTRY SONG, "Some Days are Diamonds, Some Days are Stones"? On the surface, that title may seem to be telling you that some days are better than others, which is, as we all know, the truth. But what it's also telling you is that neither good days nor bad days stick around. Every day is different. Every day is a change. So it is with you, too.

Acceptance of yourself is part of your foundation as a writer and a human being. I know it sounds like a trite New Age concoction of the week, but stick with me for a minute. Being able to look at yourself with unflinching honesty and a hint of a smile is going to give you something real to work with. Building yourself up beyond what you are currently capable of or tearing yourself down won't serve you. Humans are perfectly imperfect. If you can't honestly acknowledge the areas you can work on, then you won't do any work; conversely, if you don't honestly acknowledge your strengths, you'll spend your energy working on what is already strong.

Some of us came from backgrounds in which it was impolite or even sinful to brag, and we equate acknowledging our strengths as bragging. Bragging is what occurs when you tear others down to build yourself up. Standing straight and strong in the truth of who you are is not bragging; it's honesty. Some of us can't acknowledge what we're good at. We blush, deflect, and point out a huge flaw in ourselves when we're given a compliment.

"You look great in that shirt," our friend says.

"Oh, this? I got it for a buck at Goodwill. It's just junk."

Practice accepting compliments. Practice giving them to yourself. It also helps to practice giving them to others. Believe that you are worthy of this life you have and that you can, will, and are making positive contributions to the world.

When you see yourself realistically, you'll see your writing realistically. If we think we're perfect, we won't be able to hear helpful comments from peers on our poetry. If we think everything we do is a disaster, we won't be able to see the beauty that is hidden in the verses. Writing is an art that requires work. A writer's training is ongoing, lifelong learning. If I believe I know everything there is to know, that arrogance translates to the page, and I won't be able to actually reach a place where my work communicates effectively. If I believe I don't know anything and never will, the same result occurs.

Part of accepting who you are is accepting that you are a writer. When the memoirist Mark Spragg came to speak to a class I was teaching, he told the students that he lived the life he thought writers lived. When he read the book jackets of his favorite books, the authors were farmers or explorers or hermits. They didn't thank their MFA program or their artist colony for giving them time, space, or inspiration. They just lived their lives and then wrote about them because they were compelled to. Spragg felt like we needed to do more living and less thinking about being a writer. You are a writer or you aren't. Don't waste your effort thinking about it.

Being a writer is a way of seeing the world. It is a way of integrating the information we are in contact with every day. If you are a writer, you can no more not be a writer than you can not inhale. When you try to not be a writer, because it is too inconvenient, or you are too frightened, or you feel you are not good enough, you will notice this repression of your authentic self surfacing in other areas. You may become addicted to something. You may find yourself growing bitter or frustrated. You may blame your personal relationships on your lack of fulfillment. Everyone has a different reason for separating themselves from their gift. But sooner or later, the gift demands to be heard. Far better for you and the rest of the world if you cultivate this relationship now. Hold writing close to your heart, whether you are writing a journal, an essay, or your memoirs for your grandchildren. It is a part of who you are, and it demands the same oxygen as any other living being. When you feed it, it feeds you. When you withhold food from it, it becomes a parasite and drains you in the most unexpected of ways. Bring writing into your life with the intimacy and regularity of brushing your teeth. Recognize it as part of who you are, not as something you *do*. It is a way of being. Absolutely nothing less will satisfy either of you.

It is hard to see ourselves accurately, and just as hard to see our work accurately. That's one of the reasons writers have groups or colleagues who read and respond to their work. They know they can't see it all and want some honest assessment. The longer you practice your craft, the more objectively you'll be able to see your work. You'll get better over time. Objectivity is an essential skill so a writer can effectively revise and analyze his work. You can't do it if you can't detach from it and see it objectively and honestly.

Every day you sit down to write is a different day than the day before. You're a different person than the day before. Different triggers are pushed. Different memories are floating around. Different sensations are in the body. When the writing is going well, notice, smile softly, and carry on. When the writing isn't going so well, notice, smile softly, and carry on.

When you fight where you are, you create resistance and tension in the body and the mind. If the writing isn't going well and you start to rant and rave, tighten your jaw and your shoulders, shorten your breath, you're giving energy to the *fight* and you're ensuring that the work is going to stay stuck because you're focused on the stuckness rather than the impermanence of this particular writing day. Show up tomorrow and it will be different. Decide you have a block and don't want to play anymore, and you'll surely have that block and you won't be a writer and you'll have given your power to the impermanence of the moment of yesterday. Don't do it.

I know it's tempting. If you read memoirs by writers or other books about the writing life, you'll see a consistent mention of the need to keep your butt in the chair. Every writer finds her own way to work with the resistances and the bad days, because in order to live this path, you have to find that way. You begin to feel (not rationalize) that when you keep your butt in the chair, eventually something appears. When you don't show up, or when you walk away at the first moment of discomfort, not too much appears. When you learn to accept the days of less flexibility, fewer words on the paper, more rambling, you're building your foundation for the days of great flexibility, surprising phrases and concepts, and focused pieces. Treat your writing as an integral part of your life and the ebbs and flows of your relationship with it won't seem as startling or as severe. Some days you and your friend seem like you're speaking in alternate universes. Some days you and your writing will seem the same.

Recognize your limitations, but don't make them life sentences. Instead of saying, "I can't write in iambic pentameter," say, "I can't write in iambic pentameter *today*." And then, if iambic pentameter is what you seek, read it, practice it, tomorrow is another day. Without the work (the reading and the practicing), you'll be saying the same thing tomorrow. A new day doesn't bring you a wondrous new set of skills without work. Accepting where you need to work allows you to build a foundation that is solid, not pockmarked with delusions about your current abilities. The lesson of impermanence teaches us that whatever we're currently feeling will pass. The lesson of acceptance allows us to find joy in every part of the writing process.

Touchstones

1. Write a love letter to yourself. You can write it from any point of view you like. You might experiment with different points of view. For example, one letter might come from you to yourself, one from your lover to you, one from a character in your book, etc.

2. Make a list of your writing strengths and weaknesses. What can you do to work on your areas of weakness? Be specific with your ideas. Don't just say, "Read more." Find books that focus on your weakness. For example, if you feel you're weak on dialogue, you might read David Mamet or Alice Walker. Check out how they do it. If you're weak on setting, read James Agee's *A Death in the Family* or Larry McMurtry's *Lonesome Dove*. If you think you're weak on

characterization, try Toni Morrison's *Beloved* or Sena Jeter Naslund's *Four Spirits*. Expand your experience.

3. Try writing a bragging poem about anything at all you do well or love about yourself. Pull out all the stops. Don't be afraid of sounding arrogant. Tell the world about how wonderful you are. And laugh!

7

RELATIONSHIP

Piglet sidled up to Pooh from behind. "Pooh!" he whispered.
"Yes, Piglet?"
"Nothing," said Piglet, taking Pooh's paw. "I just wanted to make sure of you."

A. A. MILNE

EACH NEW SEMESTER, a number of students return to the classroom after they've crossed a major life threshold such as divorce or retirement. Many of them took a creative writing class decades ago and are frustrated because now that *they* are ready, they are confused about why they aren't churning out books like Stephen King. It took me awhile to figure out what was at the heart of this type of student's problems. It wasn't that they weren't smart enough or well-read enough. It was that they hadn't maintained and nurtured a relationship with their writing over the years, so it had, quite simply, quit waiting around for them to show up.

Every writer has a unique relationship to his or her writing, and it is in the dynamics of this relationship that the perils, joys, and challenges of a writer's life breathe. Precisely because writing is not often approached as a *relationship,* but rather a task to be completed or a goal to be met, writers run into unexpected problems that they didn't find mentioned in their texts on writing solid dialogue or creating characters that jump off the page.

Think back to your ten- or twenty-year high school reunion. If you're too young for that, think about a friend you've lost contact with. What happens if you run into that person unexpectedly? That person might have been the love of your life at fifteen, but twenty years later you find yourselves staring at each other over the punch bowl wondering how you ever had a conversation at all. Why? The obvious reason is that you haven't worked to maintain that relationship, and so the gap between you is too difficult to bridge.

It is no different with your writing. You either form and maintain and nurture a relationship with your writing, or every time you return to the page, you'll be starting from the beginning—the "what's your sign?" level of conversation. When you set out on the writer's path, set out with the same level of commitment that you have with your partner or children or best friend. Don't take this trip partway. You'll find yourself frustrated, angry at the writing. You'll hear the most misused words in a writing class slip past your lips. "The writing just isn't there!" But the truth of that statement is *you* haven't been there. How long would you wait alone at a restaurant for your date to show up? Writing is no different.

A common lament among my students in my writing classes is that they do not have enough time to finish/start/ commit to their projects. I hear lots of "When I finish raising my kids . . ." or "When I retire . . ." or even "When I win the lottery . . ." types of sentences. The structure of these sentences implies that writing is something to do at some point in the future, when all the planets have aligned. They imply that writing is only an external activity that can be worked on in a single large chunk at the end of our lives.

There are several flaws in this logic. First, despite all our time-saving devices, many of us feel like we have less time than ever before. That's not true, though. We have the same time as we've always had. It's our perception of that time that has gotten off balance. We haven't shortened the day or the hour; we have increased what we're filling that time with, and for many of us, what we fill the hours with are distractions from the very thing we say we want more of—a present moment. Rather than say, "I don't have any time!" which is not a true statement, reevaluate your relationship to that time. How aware are you of the time you are in right now? How consciously do you fill the hours? We don't know that we'll ever reach that "nirvana" place where all the bills are paid, the kids are gone, and our health is good. We don't know that we will even have tomorrow.

Second, imagine saying, "I'm going to join the New York Philharmonic as soon as my last child is through college." Then imagine showing up for the auditions, pulling your violin from its case after having played it once or twice a year for the past twenty years, and expecting to get first chair. What are the odds? But for some reason, people tend to think that they can write a novel all at once, perfectly, sell it, make a million dollars, and retire in the Bahamas without a consistent lifelong writing practice. It's illogical thinking. The only time that exists is this moment. Write. Now.

Another way we harm our relationship to writing is by searching outside ourselves for answers. We attend seminars and conferences. We network with "real" writers, or we spend more money than we make on books that promise success in six months. Far too often, we end up with a shelf full of dusty books, credit card debt, and self-loathing over our failure to glean the magic writing formula from all our efforts.

I have seen these students appear with stacks of manuscript pages that they are both attached to and repelled by. They look to me for the magic writing formula, and some drop the class when I don't pretend to have one. The tragedy, to me, of this outward seeking, is that many of these frustrated writers are very talented. They have valuable, needed perspectives on the world. Many even know they are talented. Yet, still they flounder. When students ask questions about how to do something, and I tell them I do not know, I can see the inner monologue: *She's the teacher! How can she not know the answer?* But writing isn't math. There are no answers, except for the ones that reveal themselves to you on your own path.

Learning to write strong dialogue without a rooted foundation in your relationship to your work is like expecting your once-a-month scale practice on the piano to be enough to get you on tour with George Winston. Yes, it's possible. But it's highly unlikely. Craft is very important, of course, and I don't mean to diminish the importance of being able to form logical sentences, build tension within a scene, or organize a story structure. But it's not enough, and it is the realization that theory alone will not a writer make that frustrates students and eventually, brings them to a crisis point in their work. From this crisis point, a new way of thinking can emerge, which allows them to move away from the rules and limitations of the mind into the vast playground of the body and heart.

Many writers who reach this point think graduate school is a solution. But earning a Master of Fine Arts degree in creative writing does not mean you have mastered anything other than two years of a graduate program. You will likely find more tools at your disposal, and you will have demonstrated a commitment to your work, but you won't find a writing key for all your writing woes. There is no key that unlocks the mysteries of what your writing is to you. Once you solve one puzzle, another one reveals itself. Once you find your way through a sticky plot construction or a research question or a dialogue issue, all you have done is resolved that particular problem. You've not solved all future plot problems. You've not uncovered the holy grail of your writing. You cannot will your writing to appear and disappear on demand. You can, through disciplined practice, cultivate a relationship with it that allows you both to thrive, but if you sit down at the keyboard and order, "Write!" at 3 a.m., your likely result will be forced words, if any appear at all. Think about how well *you* respond when ordered to do something. Your writing is the same way. Treat it as you would like to be treated.

I really encourage you to think about your writing practice as a relationship. Cultivate a respect for each other. Just as in any of your human relationships, maintain healthy boundaries. Don't let yourself become so enmeshed in your writing that you measure your life by its rhythms. There's a whole world out there. You should probably experience some of it so that when you return to your desk you'll have something to write about.

It's healthy to *not* write from time to time as well. Take breaks from each other. Kahlil Gibran says, "Let there be spaces in your togetherness." This is as true with writing as it is with people. I don't encourage you to take a several-year sabbatical, but if you do, recognize that you'll return not just to a computer or notebook, but to a relationship. Treat it as such and don't expect things to pick up right where you left off. This is less frightening to do if you've already made space for it. The writer who screams, "I can't take a break from it!

I can't even get myself to sit down three times a week!" hasn't cleared out the closet for the writing to move in. This is a live-in relationship. You can't just date and hope to keep the spark alive over a lifetime. Make space in your life for it. Don't just give it half of the underwear drawer. Give it room to breathe and grow and surprise you. Don't chain it up and tell it what kind of stories to write or what rhyme schemes to use. Mutual respect and trust will go a long way.

This may sound ridiculous, but what I'm trying to show you is a way to move from the abstract to the concrete (something we do all the time in writing) with your writing life too. The more specific you can be with everything, the more rewarding your attempts will be. Personify writing and make it a character in your life. It's great practice and will also help you move into a relationship with it. Just as it's hard for the reader to connect when the author uses too many abstract ideas, it's hard for you to connect to your writing if it's just some abstract idea or ideal "out there" somewhere. Bring it into your house. Find out what size jeans it wears. Does it prefer coffee or tea? It's an equal relationship, not a relationship built on the hierarchy of you as boss or it as master. Seek that in-between space in all your doings.

Like any relationship, there will be bumps, places where you don't communicate very well, places where you are irritated by everything that occurs. If you see these times through the lens of relationship, then you'll be less likely to cry "foul" and quit writing. There are phases to everything. Embrace what each phase has to teach you, knowing it is impermanent.

The second level of relationship with your work applies to the individual projects you're working on. Each character in your novel is a relationship you form. You experience their journeys *with* them; you don't inflict their journeys *on* them. The more you read and the more you write, the more you'll begin to feel (not think) the stories. You'll start to feel which plot turns are cheesy and which ones are innovative. You'll start to feel when you're working with caricatures, rather than characters. But you won't know by thinking it. You'll know by *feeling*. Meet your characters with an open heart, curiosity, humility, and acceptance. Then, pick up your pen and listen.

Few experiences match the joy that arises when we capture that perfect combination of words to express what we are feeling. Endorphins are released. We sit back in our chairs with absolute awe. We are infatuated with our work. Over time, the infatuation matures and we see both our strengths and shortcomings. We recognize that a deep relationship with our writing depends upon us being able to embrace equally what we do well and what we do not do well. Accepting this paradox brings joy. When the relationship is entered into joyfully, it produces work of a quality and content we could not have imagined. If we trust the writing process, we will be repaid over and over again by this deepening relationship. We show up to the page and the writing shows up to the page. Writing sustains us when the world around us is crumbling. Like a favorite pair of jeans, it surrounds us with flawed comfort, durability, flexibility, and security.

Touchstones

1. Write a poem or story or letter to your writing. Personify the writing if you like.

2. Take your protagonist out to lunch. Take your notebook and plan a "date" with him or her. Where would she like to go? What would she like to eat? What movie would he like to see? Use this time as a chance to revel in the relationship between you and your characters.

3. Interview your character. You can use a traditional journalistic approach or be casual and informal.

4. Create a silly "relationship" quiz like the kind found in fashion magazines to chart your relationship with your writing. Play! What do you notice?

5. Create a space in your house for your writing. It doesn't have to be a whole room. Just a table, or corner of the house that is only for you and your writing. It might take time for you to find the right location, but it's worth it. It honors both you and the work.

6. Create internal space for your writing. Use your journal to uncover where there is room inside you for your writing to breathe. Discover what is crowding its space, what could be discarded, and what could be added.

7. Wine and dine your writing. Do something concrete to "woo" it. How can you keep the romance alive in the long term?

PART TWO

THE DEEP WRITING PROCESS

Opportunity is missed by most people
because it is dressed in overalls and looks like work.

THOMAS EDISON

The cycle of our breathing sustains our lives. We complete this cycle over 25,000 times per day. This consistency of breath—inhale, pause, exhale, pause—is our body's engine. The consistency of our writing practice will sustain the heart of our writing lives. We must show up and put pen to paper over and over and over again, whether we feel inspired or not.

In part 2, we'll address the craft of writing. When you don't pay attention to how scenes are sculpted, how point of view works, or how to best punctuate your sentences, the result is sloppy writing. Your inattention to detail is disrespectful to your readers and your art. Here, we'll discuss the key components of a story, poem, or memoir that are essential to creating a solid, accessible piece of writing. Now is the time to take your beautiful and brilliant stream of consciousness journal entries and accept them for what they are: stream of consciousness journal entries. Continue further inward now. Recognize, with humility, that there is still a lot of work to be done. A lot of shaping, revising, fine-tuning. But you've got the heart to work with now. Without that, you'd be fine-tuning nothing.

Part 2 will also help you find ways to embrace the work itself. The trial and error. The false starts. The interminable discovery phase. The relentless precision of the revision. A serious writer knows that writing takes, well, writing. A serious writer knows that it is through the working and reworking of the material that it begins to breathe. A serious writer knows that she is not infallible. That the words that drip from her pen are not perfect the first (or second, or third) time out.

The hardest piece for many writers is actually the "butt in chair" part of the process. For these writers, it is far more enjoyable to talk about the things they are *going* to write, or

Body Break

You may find yourself agitated during the working stage. Or, you may find yourself needing some inspiration and energy. Try this:

1. If you need to calm your mind, lie on the floor on your right side and breathe deeply. This will naturally cause gravity to slightly close off the right nostril, which will result in an increase of oxygen in the left nostril. This will help cool your mind.
2. If you need to stimulate your body or writing process, lie on the floor on your left side and breathe deeply. This will naturally cause gravity to slightly close off the left nostril, which will result in an increase of oxygen in the right nostril. This will help warm your body and increase your energy flow.

plan for the life that will be theirs *after* they write. But of course, in order to reach the point where you hold a book of your own in your hands, you must do more than talk about writing and dream about the National Book Award. You must sit down, pick up the pen or open the laptop, and begin stringing words together.

This section will help you find the threads to hang your words on.

8

SELF-AWARENESS

In the world to come, I shall not be asked, "Why were you not Moses?"
I shall be asked, "Why were you not Zusya?"

RABBI ZUSYA

SELF-AWARENESS IS THE PRIMARY foundational principle of deep writing. Self-awareness is important because when you see yourself and your world from a place of nonjudgment and honesty, you can clearly see the areas you need to work on in your writing. If you don't have a realistic picture (or refuse to look at one) of your strengths and weaknesses, you'll likely flounder longer than you need to. *Every* writer has strengths and weaknesses. No writer is perfect at all the components of writing. Acknowledge and honor the strengths and weaknesses of your own writing self and you'll be well on the way to deepening your craft.

It's human nature to play to our strengths. If we're really good with dialogue, we will likely use a lot of it. If we're not so good with plotting, we will find ourselves drawn to writing character-based pieces. This is natural. But in order to grow, we have to move into places of discomfort. We have to learn to swim just as easily in the oceans of plotting as we do in the rivers of dialogue. One of your tasks is to honestly assess which part of the writing process you most resonate with and which part you'd rather gnaw off your fingers than work with.

Let's look at the basic writing process. The key word is *process*. Writing requires steps. Any English 101 textbook will outline these basics. Terminology varies slightly from book to book, but we can essentially break it all down into two main parts: prewriting and revising.

Prewriting is also called brainstorming, freewriting, discovering, questioning, bubbling, and any number of "ing" words. This is the place of discovery. This is where we are truly free, unencumbered, and outside of our ego's control. We can write in a stream-of-consciousness style. We don't have to worry about pesky things like grammar and syntax. We don't have to use paragraphs. In this place, everything we write has the possibility of being the step that leads us to the next level. Prewriting also includes the first draft of your piece. Here, the world is rosy, perfect, and full of wonder. This is where we rant, make false starts, figure out who our characters are, and surprise ourselves.

Prewriting is a receptive place. It involves listening, stepping back, opening up. Everything is lovely. We are energized about our ideas. We have passion for our characters and a drive to discover the story. There's a "rush" in this stage. A fire. We can't wait to start writing and we wish we could spend all our days in this space of awe and amazement. For every writer who loves this stage, there is a writer who feels like he's being skinned alive with all this meandering.

Know this: The writer who remains in the prewriting stage may end up with drawers full of journals that have helped her personal growth tremendously, but she won't have a publishable novel or poem. She'll have a foundation, but not a polished piece. The writer who thinks her work is perfect just as it is, just as she wrote it the very first time, is not a writer.

The second part of the writing process is the revisioning stage, which encompasses several steps. This is the time when we get to engage our left brains. We take a step back, read our drafts with a critical eye, and begin shaping and sculpting them using the tools of our craft so that the heart we uncovered in the prewriting phase can become something the reader can connect with.

This energy is active, full of *doing*, and sometimes it is ruthless in its cutting and paring away. It's work. Here, we take that fire we had popping and sizzling all over the place in the prewriting stage and douse it with water. Only the strongest burns with the richest fuel sources keep going. We may grow to hate our work because it didn't turn out like we wanted it. We may get bored with it. The nuts-and-bolts nature of this stage is precision work. It is also very exciting and stimulating, and yes, there's still discovery to be had. But it is work. Likely, the writers who loved the prewriting phase are now digging their heels in with resistance to this part of the process.

Here, we do as many drafts as it takes to get the work to a place where it actually works. A common question at writers' conferences is, "How many drafts did you go through?" There is no single correct answer for this, as each project dictates its own needs. It takes as many drafts as it takes. The only guarantee is that it takes more than one draft. Always. Write this down somewhere and post it prominently over your workspace. *The first draft is only the beginning.*

The revisioning stage is when we step back and see our work with fresh eyes. We begin again, with a strong foundation underneath us. We have solid footing, so things begin to take shape. We get to really use all the tools of our craft we've been learning about. The more we read with the eyes of a writer, the better we'll be at helping our own work at this step. Here's where knowing all the ramifications of point-of-view choices will come in handy. Here's where you decide whether to use interpolated or modulated dialogue. Here's where you create the pacing and the tension and where you create your concrete images. This is also the step where you edit and proofread. You tighten the sentences until they sing. You fine-tune your word choices. You remove needless words.

Know this: If a writer only does this part, he will still not have a publishable work. He may have a series of grammatically correct sentences, but the heart will be missing. The writer who spends his days agonizing over the opening sentence when he only has three sentences will spend his days in opening sentences.

Ultimately, the goal is to write from a place of union. We want to bring these active and receptive components together. It's not an either/or relationship. It is a both/and one. If you love freewriting and journaling, that's wonderful. But know that the area you need to work on is the drafting and polishing process. You need to be just as excited about the craft issues and the sentence level choices. If you love working a sentence until it is as good as it can be, that's also great. Make sure you spend some time in the uncharted waters of freewriting. Swim in both oceans. The work will be richer for it.

Here are some questions you might consider as you ponder the notion of self-awareness. What drives you to write? In other words, why on earth do you want to do this instead of watching the game and eating a bag of potato chips? As I sit here in my office looking out at the tops of piñon pines, I can't think of a good reason that would either compel you to pick up the book or compel me to write it. I can't imagine why anyone would pay me to do such a thing. My mind/ego starts to get a handle on things pretty strongly at this point and I start tearing myself apart. Does my agent have any idea how bad I am at committing and finding time for my own work? Does she know how many ways I procrastinate, how much effort I spend to avoid this thing that I say I love? Do I actually love it, or do I do it because I have no other choice? Wouldn't it be great to plop down on the couch and turn on the TV and veg the night away? On more than one occasion I've wished I could do that. On more than one occasion I've wished I could shut off this drive in me—but fortunately this doesn't last very long, because, if I think it through, I end up with these deeper questions:

> What would I do then?
> What would I do without this voice calling inside me?
> Who would I be without it?
> How much does writing define who you are? Or, maybe a better question—how much does *not* writing define who you are?

I always look at my new crop of creative writing students each year and think—wow, how brave they are. They have answered the call to write—what perhaps they don't know—but they know there's some drive inside them that they need to pay attention to. And they are fighting the voices of practicality to show up. They are battling their own hopes. They haven't figured out yet that they didn't show up to *do* something. They showed up to *listen* to something deeper inside them than they thought possible. This is a tricky place. The mind/ego raises nasty questions: How are you going to make a living? What do you have to say that matters? The world won't care. No one gets published anymore. You're wasting your time when you could be doing (fill in the blank). These demons have to be battled before deep writing can occur. You can look at them one by one, just like you write one word before the other. Then, they don't have nearly so much power.

Writing is so much more than picking up a pen—but of course, that is what it ultimately is. We first must address what is in the way of the path between our hearts and our paper. Writing and the benefits of writing are available to anyone, whether publication is a goal or not. Writing, in addition to a form of communication, is also reflection and thinking. When we write, we give ourselves pause before we react. We can problem solve, both personally and globally.

Really take a moment to consider why you write. One way to think about this question is to flip it around. Try to identify what *is* there by identifying what is missing. If you examine honestly the reason why you don't write (or procrastinate or avoid the act of writing), you will find clues to why it is so important for you to do so. Go ahead. Just try. It's in your process journal. No one ever has to see it.

Touchstones

1. Are you your writing? Who (or what) are you? Who does the writing? Begin with a clean slate. Just for a moment (and you can tell your ego it's just an exercise), give in to the notion that you are empty. You are a hollow chamber for breath. Sit with that image. You're clean. Clear. No baggage from the past. No desires for the future. You're pure and perfect. Start here. Freewrite for fifteen minutes.

2. Write a descriptive piece showing your life if you were not writing. Be very specific—what is there? What isn't there? Try to avoid vague "feeling" words like "sad, empty, lonely." Instead, show how those feelings (or whatever feelings relate to you) are manifested in your scene.

3. What do you believe is the inherent value in poetry? In novels? In literature? What do you believe is important about it? How does literature make you feel? Journal about it for fifteen minutes.

9

PROCESS VS. PRODUCT

The purpose of a fish trap is to catch fish, and when the fish are caught, the trap is forgotten. The purpose of a rabbit snare is to catch rabbits. When the rabbits are caught, the snare is forgotten. The purpose of words is to convey ideas. When the ideas are grasped, the words are forgotten. Where can I find a man who has forgotten words? He is the one I would like to talk to.

CHUANG-TZU

THE LONGER I TEACH CREATIVE WRITING, the more apparent the need to emphasize process over product becomes to me. Perhaps because our culture is intently focused on products, end results, outcomes assessment. If I had a dollar for every student who came by my office three days before final grades were due and asked what he or she could do to pass the class, I'd retire wealthy. It's become more important to get a grade than to mature as a writer. Likewise, I notice writers, especially beginning writers, focusing on an end product. They ask marketing questions. They ask about finding an agent and a publisher. They ask about advance money and book tours and Oprah. They rarely read. They haven't written a novel yet, or even a short story that holds together. But they have an outcome, and the outcome drives them, rather than the art itself. I tell them the product doesn't matter, not at this point in their writing development, but I know they don't believe me. At eighteen, I don't think I would have believed me. Once they begin publishing, they will see that the work doesn't change. It's still there. Publication didn't dramatically change their lives, make them a better person, shower them with wealth beyond their wildest dreams, or bring about world peace. With any luck, they might begin to think maybe publication isn't what it's all about.

If you hold on to the goal of publication as the hallmark for your success as a writer, you are giving away your power. Obviously, most of us who write want to be published because we are trying to communicate with others. We are attempting to connect. But most of the publishing process is out of our control. Trends change. Editors leave. Magazines start up and fold. There are no guarantees. And, when we *do* get published, nothing of substance in our lives has changed. We still have only our relationship with the blank page. We still have new material. The same anxieties we had before publication don't miraculously vanish. If we have attached our personal success or failure to an outcome of publication, we have set ourselves up to be continually looking into the future and judging our present actions against something that is completely out of our control. In short, we have set ourselves up to suffer.

I write because I can't *not* write. I do want to communicate, and I want the work I love to find a home in the world, but if it never did, if I had never sold a book or story or essay in my life, I would still write. I know this because there were many years where I didn't do any of those things, yet still I wrote. The writing outlasts jobs, partners, and pets. The writing itself is the continuum of our lives. The writing is not a task to be accomplished; it is a relationship to be nurtured and cultivated throughout our lives.

I realize how ridiculous it sounds for someone who has published to advise you not to worry about publication. Sure, easy for me to say, right? But please understand I am not telling you *not* to publish. I'm simply suggesting that you write. Write whenever you can. Write when you're too tired to write. Write even when you're convinced you've written the most brilliant thing in the world or when you have nothing to say or too much to say. And when you're not writing, read. If you keep up this pattern of writing and reading, publication will be much more easily attained. You'll have the tools to do the work, and the work will become a way of life for you. You'll see that publication is as fickle as the weather. But you'll keep on writing. That's the constant, and that's the space you stand in.

Seeking balance between goal setting and a tra-la-la land of meandering is a challenge every writer faces. I think it is important to have a direction, sort of a loose plan, if you will, for your writing life. The danger I see in hard and fast goals is that the idea of success depends upon achieving goals which you may or may not have any control over. You can't control trends in publishing. No one in publishing foresaw 9/11 and the changes that event wrought on the types of books published and, more importantly, purchased.

The key to this dilemma is unique to every individual because the solution resides in the relationship you have with yourself. How well do you know your own habits and patterns? How well do you operate under pressure? What do you use pressure to achieve in your life? How focused are you on achieving?

Likely, you fall into one of three camps: One, you set lots

of goals and are very driven to achieve them. As soon as you do achieve them, you set lots more goals. You're always reaching. Or two, you set lots of goals, don't achieve them or fall short of them in some way, and get frustrated and decide you can't do anything. Or three, you never set any goals and just let whatever happens happen, resulting in a lot of started projects but very few finished ones. Don't worry; you're not a bad person or a doomed writer if you recognize parts of yourself in these camps. You're human. Writing is just like any other job. You have to show up for it. We're almost pre-programmed to set goals in America. We set deadlines for ourselves so we'll *do* something. This is fine, but recognize that you're tricking yourself into giving yourself motivation to *do the work*. I think you'll find your writing will open up when you find a way to do the work regardless of any goal.

I want to emphasize that I am not telling you to never set goals or never hope to achieve things in your life. I'm simply hoping you'll allow for the possibility of a new way of thinking that will allow you to shift your energy away from a constant seeking and channel that energy into a consistent practice. It's what you do now that will allow you to have the future you're seeking.

Suppose your rooftop needs some maintenance. A windstorm has ripped off some shingles. You can't put it off anymore. It's time to climb on the roof and take care of the mess. What's the goal? To fix the shingles, right? What do you need to get on the roof? A ladder. Think of a ladder like an intention. For example, I'm coming to a writing class because I want to get published. OK, that's great. That intention gets you out the door and into class (or onto the roof). But once you get on the roof, you don't pull the ladder up with you. You have to release the ladder in order to get the work done on the shingles (unless you've got six or seven hands!).

It's the same with writing. It's OK if a desire for publication is what gets you in the chair doing the work. Whatever gets you there is fine. But once you get there, let it go. Let yourself be with your work. The desire will dance in front of you, ever more seductively, if you let it in, and rather than be a cheerleader pulling you forward toward your goal, it will spin you in circles until you no longer remember why you sat down to write or what you hoped to say. You've been dancing with desire, and you're tired now. The writing can wait. Desire has won.

I know of no writer, myself included, who hasn't had to learn how to manage desire. Desire can be lots of things. It doesn't have to be a desire for publication (which could keep you endlessly searching the Internet or *Poets & Writers* magazine for places you could *send* your work rather than allowing you to *do* the work). It could be a thirst for companionship. A need to spend money. To eat too much food. To indulge in anything that keeps you from staying put, butt in chair, writing. I actually purchased my laptop computer because I found that the Internet (and all the shopping potential there) was my "dancing desire." It was way too easy to sit down at the computer with the intention of working for two hours only to find myself sucked into a never-ending field of cute clothes and amazing books. So, I have to write at a computer that's not hooked up to the web. I've learned to trick myself, and the irony of purchasing something to avoid purchasing something has not escaped me. But it's a way I manage.

Maybe you like to chat online. Maybe you like to garden or talk on the phone or watch soap operas. None of these activities is intrinsically bad. The secret lies in how and why you do them. If you come to a yoga class because you want to lose weight or become more flexible, there's nothing wrong with that. But once you walk in the door of the class, leave those reasons at the door and just *be in the class.* Flexibility and weight loss will occur over time because you're showing up for the work. Writing is just like that. Keep showing up. It'll take you places you never thought possible.

Touchstones

1. Describe your writing process. What other areas of your life are similar in their process nature? Find a specific image for your writing process when it is in flow. Find another specific image for your writing process when it is not in flow. Can these two images dialogue with each other? What are the gifts of each of the images?

2. What are the obstacles on your path? These can be physical objects or emotional obstacles or anything in between. Write them down. You might make a map of the obstacles. Have fun exploring your own mind's ability to complicate things. Remember, when you can see it and name it, you take away its power.

3. Bonnie Friedman, in her book *Beyond the Words,* talks about *percolation* as being an important part of the writing process. This is the time to explore and let ideas germinate. How do you experience percolation? How do you distinguish it from laziness or avoidance of the story? Do you?

10

BODY AS SOURCE

Oh, darling, let your body in, let it tie you in,
in comfort.

ANNE SEXTON

I DON'T REMEMBER THE DAY I first moved out of my body. Sometime in childhood the detachment began. The criticism of a waist not as slim as the other girls, of breasts bigger, legs shorter. The frustration with not being able to run or jump as fast or high as the others. The transition I made from body to brain was subtle, like the shifting of the tectonic plates, so slow as not to be noticeable until suddenly an ocean is where a desert once was. Other kids wanted to run, play sports, climb trees. I wanted to curl up inside and write and read. Outside was best viewed through double paned glass. I felt that way about my body, too. It was best viewed at a distance, useful as a vehicle to carry my brain around, but that was about all. What was important was that I could think, communicate, talk, learn, teach. It wasn't nearly so important that I be able to move.

In 1995, I was living in Phoenix and working in marketing. One Saturday I stopped for a quick drive-through meal. When

I began driving home, everything went black. I didn't pass out. I was conscious. I was driving. It wasn't just that dizziness that everyone gets from time to time where the world gets blurry and shifts directions. I saw black. My heart rate escalated, a tachycardia rhythm I'd experienced since early childhood. I don't know how long the world was dark. Long enough for me to envision the traffic accident I was about to cause. My vision returned, but my right arm had been weakened. My grip, once strong, couldn't grasp another's hand and squeeze. I was twenty-seven and suddenly realized my body mattered. It wasn't just a shell to house a mind, it was its own *thing*—a creature that I was inside every minute of my life and had no knowledge of. A creature that might have an agenda different from my own. Or perhaps, one that was mine all along.

Doctors couldn't find anything other than the tachycardia, which had always been there. They suggested pills. I didn't want pills. I wanted to know this body, not medicate it. I didn't want to shut it up anymore or be in conflict with it anymore. How to do that? How to move into my own skin? I started off doing step aerobics, where I quickly learned that trying to force my way into my body and take over (acting like I'd been there all along) was a surefire way to get injured. This is when I found my way into a yoga class, where I've stayed ever since.

Yoga is slow. Mindful. It cultivates a relationship between body, mind, and spirit, but it requires discipline and commitment to feel the benefits. Yoga isn't a thirty-day fix to whatever ails you. But as I worked with yoga, I began to listen, for the first time, to my body. Yes, that feels good. No, that stretch is too deep, pull back. I noticed sudden tears surfacing during a spinal twist and the incredible, surprising unburdening (of what?) that occurred in pigeon pose. I began to welcome conversations between me and this form of flesh that carries me.

When I truly began to listen to my own skin, I could hardly contain the din. It was like a mother coming home from work to a dozen kids all talking at once. It panicked me, being this close to my skin. No wonder we distract ourselves from it in every conceivable way. This skin, this body, held *everything* I'd ever done. Through showing up on the mat, I learned to show up for my body. My ability, not just to listen, but to hear, surfaced. And as I learned how to hear, I learned how to write in a new way.

By moving into a different place inside myself, my relationship to my writing also shifted. The slower I moved, the deeper I moved. The same effect emerged in the writing. The slower I wrote, meaning the longer I lingered in a scene, the more was revealed to me about the scene. The more I stayed with whatever was surfacing, the more I discovered what I was really writing about. We have to linger, staying with discomfort long enough to name it, embrace it, and integrate it. Lingering awhile gives your work the space it needs to bloom. Conscious breathing helps create this space. Our breath directs our awareness. Follow our breath and we find ourselves.

Being in the body is the first step toward being "grounded," having your feet on the earth. But before your characters can be on the earth, they must be *of body*. They cannot be only of mind and thoughts. If they are only thoughts, you've got lots of roaming eyeballs and abstract ideas appearing in your work. You've got to put your characters in a body, and no, the body is not yours.

Accessing our physical bodies and consequently the bodies of our characters is another piece of the deep-writing puzzle. Bodies are much more than the muscles of our fingers and wrists. Bodies are grounded in a physical world, whether that world is another planet or Toledo. Bodies have needs and desires that may be at odds with the character's current desires. Notice how even when you are focused writing a scene, you still have a throbbing ankle, or an itchy ear, or an ache in your right shoulder. So do your characters. You still hear the noise from the wannabe musician next door or the hum of the heater on the roof. You hear the soft snoring of your ancient cat. Remember: we do not leave this world to write another world. It's through living in this world completely that we are able to write those other worlds.

A particularly bookish, awkward student of mine spends every spare minute in class reading a thick book. His glasses are equally thick, as is his body. I watched him walk from class to the Student Union one day, and his head was quite literally a foot in front of his body. He walked at an angle, his head leading the way, legs struggling to catch up. Many writers live in their heads. They flee to their imaginations and they don't always notice the rest of their bodies. When I saw the physical manifestation of the schism between this student's head and his body, I was reminded of how physically present a writer must be to merge with his or her stories. I was reminded of how small, proportionately, our heads are compared to the rest of our bodies. Deep writing requires presence in your whole being, whatever it looks like, whatever its limitations. Move into your body and you will move into your writing.

I remember when I was about eight being carried on the shoulders of my very tall uncle. I could see the dust on top of the refrigerator! I remember being amazed that he was as tall as the top of the refrigerator, and I recognized *through my own body* how differently he viewed the world from me, and that that difference was partly based on where his head was in relationship to the earth. My father had polio as a boy and never fully regained the use of his left leg. His worldview was partly shaped through his weakened leg. I have worn very thick

Body Break

Put the book down and place your hands together, palm to palm in front of you. Allow your hands to open, like the cover of a book. Separate them as slowly as you can. Notice how it feels when skin touches skin, and how it feels when separation occurs. Open and close this book of your body as many times as you like.

glasses, and later contact lenses, since second grade. I don't remember being able to see clearly the outlines of leaves and blades of grass with my own eyes. I don't remember ever waking up and seeing precisely the room I was in. My worldview is partly shaped through nearsightedness. When you create characters, ask yourself:

What bodies do your characters inhabit?
Where are their scars?
Where did they skin their knees or break their
  bones or suffer from a blood disease?
How are their bodies marked by their lives?
What emotional traumas have taken up residence
  in their lungs or joints or (fill in the blank)?

I used to wonder when I was a girl why none of the characters in the books I read ever had to go to the bathroom. Now, I realize that those things are not generally essential to the plot of the story, so they don't get included, but I remember thinking it was really odd that none of these fictional beings had to do any of the day-to-day "body things" that I had to do. Did they ever itch? Have oily hair? Stinky armpits? Rogue hairs that pop out on their chins? *You* need to know these things about your characters, whether or not they make it into the final manuscript. You need to know them because if you give your characters bodies—give them feet to move around the earth on—they'll help connect your reader to the work through her cells.

Being aware of your body keeps you present. What if you never left? What if you became so aware of your breathing that you stayed, right here, right now, with your very own body in your very own life?

What if, indeed.

Touchstones

1. Choose a place of tightness in your own body to focus on for this exercise. Touch that place—not with your hands, but with your awareness. Slowly breathe into that place. Keep your awareness focused on your place of tightness and your breathing. Do you know where the tightness comes from? Can you write the story of the tension in your body? Did it come from an injury or from stress? What do you know about it? What do you *feel* about it? When you are ready, pick up your pen and write.

2. One day we will all step out of our flesh. Write a farewell letter to your body.

3. Look inward and envision your internal body. Get an anatomy book if you need to. Where are your kidneys? Liver? Lungs? Make a sketch of your internal body. Try a dialogue with a body part or a system (circulatory, respiratory, etc.). Listen to what it has to tell you.

4. Write a dialogue between you and your body. You might examine these questions: How have you failed your body? How do you feel your body has failed you? Can you find a common ground?

11

ANCESTORS AS SOURCE

And so our mothers and grandmothers have, more often than not anonymously, handed on the creative spark, the seed of the flower they themselves never hoped to see: or like a sealed letter they could not plainly read.

ALICE WALKER

WHEN I WAS JUST BEGINNING my teaching career, I attended a reading given by Joyce Carol Oates. In talking about her writing process, she mentioned the idea of writing to heal one's ancestors. I hadn't thought about writing for that purpose before, but once I heard the phrase, it was obvious to me how true it was. Writing is a way we can rewrite our stories. A way to understand the chaos of our lives and worlds. And of course, once I became aware of the concept, I saw it discussed in many different ways from many different authors across the literary canon.

We come from flesh. As science advances, we find we are able to trace our DNA back to one of ten haplogroups, which are genetic groupings of humans based on their mitochondrial DNA. The idea of interconnectedness is no longer just a New Age buzzword. We are being shown, over and over, how many ways we link together. In Anne Michaels' magical book, *Fugitive Pieces,* the narrator, Jakob Beer, is commenting on the Greek landscape he is walking through shortly after the end of World War II. He is reflecting on the horrors of the war, and says,

> Grief requires time. If a chip of stone radiates its self, its breath, so long, how stubborn might be the soul. If sound waves carry on to infinity, where are their screams now? I imagine them somewhere in the galaxy, moving forever towards the psalms.

This passage haunted me for days. I thought about the screams from every human on the planet who has suffered echoing in space forever. I thought about how much each living human being carries, not just of her own current life, but of all the lives the earth has borne witness to. I thought about the silences of my grandparents' generation, marketed as the greatest generation in part because of their stoicism. I thought about the stories their bodies held. Stories that now sleep in the earth. Where do those stories go once the last shovelful of dirt falls around the casket? Into the roots of the trees in the cemeteries? Then into the air we breathe from the photosynthesis of the trees? And then—into the nostrils of the writer walking past one spring day who suddenly hears, without a doubt, the whispering of an old man from Poland, or a Native American woman from Dakota Territory, in her ear. And then this writer, if she listens, goes home, picks up the pen, and a voice that isn't hers moves the ink.

My paternal grandmother was as closed as winter. She grew

up in the South during the Depression and made a life for herself with, as we say, spit and vinegar. She didn't talk. She, like so many of her Southern contemporaries, was a mass of contradictions. After my father died, she retreated even more inward, and when she died I was left with loose threads that made no pattern. I wanted to figure her out. I wanted to understand why she did some of the things that seemed so horrible to me. I wanted to express my deep desire to have a grandmother and all that could have been, and most of all, I wanted to forgive her and release her.

Of course, I didn't know all this when I began writing my novel, *Lay My Sorrows Down*. I had an inkling that I wanted to create a character who could give me access to my grandmother. I had a southern voice whispering to me. I wore my grandmother's engagement ring during the time I wrote that book, and when I was finished, my anger had dissipated. I was left with a human being who made choices, no different from me. In my book, the character loosely based on my grandmother is named Lillian Green. After witnessing her older brother, Tommy, lynch a black man in 1949, Lillian swallowed that secret within her. The disconnections that swim through the rest of her life are a result of her not telling her story. This is the opening paragraph from that story.

> I stopped speaking in 1949 when I was eleven years old. That was the year my older brother Tommy went crazy. The two events aren't related. Not really. It wasn't like they happened on the same day or anything. It was more like I stopped speaking and Tommy went crazy a few months later. Tommy is still crazy. He's locked up out in Mecklenburg County at one of those homes for special people. Mama wanted him to have the best, and back then

Alderman had enough to worry about, what with all the racial mess and the boys back from the war and all. Tommy doesn't seem to know he's crazy. When I go to see him, which isn't as much as I should, he's always got a big old grin on his face and he opens his arms to me and says, "Butter Bean!" Butter Bean is what he used to call me when we were growing up. I was kind of a short, round kid and one day Tommy called me Butter Bean at the supper table and it sort of stuck. Mama would never dream of calling me a frivolous name like that. To her, I was always Lillian, or sometimes Miss Lilly if I was in deep water.

This novel began with a voice, and the voice led me to circumstances, which led me to a plot, which led me to a resolution. As far as I know, my grandmother never saw a lynching, though she certainly could have, living in North Carolina most of her life. I saw a Klan rally one evening in the 1970s when we were driving home from my grandmother's house. I didn't know what it was at the time, only that my parents became very nervous and told us not to look. We all knew about the Klan, even after the sixties had passed and we were supposed to be getting along better. We all knew there were many things sleeping under the surface of the idyllic southern towns. I combined bits of what I'd seen with bits of what I knew about my grandmother and soon, Lillian became her own being, separate from me. She had her own agenda, her own reason for speaking, now that she was finally given voice. She, partly because of my own desires to uncover pieces of my own past and partly because of the interconnectedness of all of our stories, had the power not only to heal me, but also to heal others through her suffering. Writing unleashes the silenced voices.

We are able to hear them when we learn to be at ease with the silence.

The word "ancestor" means someone from whom somebody is directly descended. Sometimes we don't know who those people are. We may be one of the millions of displaced people who don't know where we came from. We may be adopted. We may be able to go back a generation but no further. We may be African descendents, or Asian descendents who came to America by force. We may be Native Americans whose pasts have been erased. It doesn't matter what skin you're walking in at this moment. What matters is who you are hearing. When you close your eyes and open your ears and your heart, who is whispering to you?

Writing is about following signposts. We don't always know what the signs are saying, only that they are somehow, some way significant. *Lay My Sorrows Down* began with a tulip image. I was going to write about a woman who grew tulips on a mist-shrouded island in the Atlantic. I researched tulips, islands, and oceans. The tulip became an important image for me as I worked through the novel, but it doesn't appear at all in the book, and Lillian neither grows tulips nor lives on an island. But each sign led to another one, like a scavenger hunt. As I released the "starter" image, I found the real image. We have to be willing to trust the signs. And, we have to be willing to discard them once we get to the next one.

Consider your own body now. What color is your skin? Be more specific than white, black, red—none of those are accurate anyway. Is your skin the color of apricot flesh? A redwood branch? The color of squirrels or pomegranates? Do you know your literal ancestry? When you look in the mirror, is it obvious where your DNA takes you back to? I am half Finnish. The other half is less easily dissected. I look Finnish, but I feel no internal connection to Finland or its people. I don't hear

Finnish voices and stories right now. But there is no doubt I carry their bloodline.

As writers we can claim a broad net for ancestors. I don't want to spend my life writing white-middle-class-female stories. I want to explore the vast sea of humanity. I want to listen for the stories that are coming to me, and I believe that if they are coming to me, then I was meant to hear them, regardless of my outer covering.

How much do you connect with your genetic ancestry? How many stories are there in each generation you can trace? Just as with all aspects of writing, look to the stories that are unspoken to find the ones with a lot of energy. Look to the moments when your aunt's lips become a straight line of silence or your cousin's eyes close for a moment longer than a blink. In those moments are stories.

Are you drawn to a culture or a time period not your own? Chances are, it's because the stories of those places intrigue you. They pique your curiosity and your writer's instincts begin to go into overdrive. They call to you—people from the Peloponnesian War, the genocide in Rwanda or Darfur, the catacombs of ancient Rome, the steppes of Russia. These voices sometimes shout, sometimes whisper, always haunt. They emerge from within and join hands with the external world. They pull you in the most unexpected places, and if you follow, you'll find signs, some written in sand, some blasting yellow neon: *You over there. Yes, I'm talking to you. You're on the right path.*

And the silent screams and joys and lives and deaths join hands with you. And as you listen to them, you change. As you hear their struggles, you change. And as you tell us all what you have learned through stories, poems, memoirs, we are all given the ability to change. And those who have gone before you lay their burdens down and move along.

Who has gone before you and laid their burdens down? Don't be afraid of where they come from. Don't be afraid that you're not worthy to tell their stories. Don't worry that they are not your gender, your religion, your sexual orientation, your ethnicity. If you hear them, they chose you, and it is your duty to answer their calls.

Touchstones

1. Where do you think your writing comes from? How does the role of the past figure into your writing? Do you think writers have a responsibility to the past? Can the past be escaped? Freewrite on these questions in your journal.

2. Listening practice. Close your eyes and imagine yourself in an empty place. Let yourself define "empty" in any way you like. Bit by bit, begin to add elements to the setting. It might be a solid redwood tree. Maybe a splashing spring. Let the setting emerge naturally, and when you feel it's complete, linger there awhile. Notice what's around you. Do you hear bees? Smell honeysuckle? Desert sage? What textures do you notice? Is the grass slick with dew? Is there a storm just to the west? Once you feel grounded in your place, be still and listen. Soon, you'll hear a voice. Trust this voice. You may only hear a sentence or you may see an entire novel. Listen. Inhale. Exhale. As you're ready, slowly open your eyes, find your pen, and begin to write.

3. Think back to a place you remember from childhood. Usually, the first place that pops into your head is the one to work with. Begin slow and small. Describe, in excruciating detail, what you see. Move through the five senses, staying as rooted to this place as you can. Find an object or area to focus on and give that object or area a voice of its own.

Yes, it's OK to personify the rocking chair. Using active listening, describe the stories that object or area tells you.

4. Make a list of time periods, historical events, people, and/or regions that interest you. When you're done, circle four of the items. Do this as fast as you can. On a new piece of paper, write down the four items from your list. Now, listen. Whose voice do you hear? You might begin with a prompt such as "I've been waiting for you" or "I didn't know how much longer I could wait before I spoke" to get the monologue moving.

12

EARTH AS SOURCE

You know they straightened out the Mississippi River in places, to make room for houses and livable acreage. Occasionally the river floods these places. "Floods" is the word they use, but in fact it is not flooding; it is remembering. Remembering where it used to be. All water has a perfect memory and is like that: remembering where it was. Writers are like that: remembering where we were, what valley we ran through, what the banks were like, the light that was there and the route back to our original place.

TONI MORRISON

THE SENSE OF PLACE IN WRITING is a basic concept taught in virtually any writing class. We need to know where we are, and we need to know who the characters are when they are in that place. Before we can do that, we must have an idea of what our own relationship to the earth is. This relationship has shifted significantly for many of us in the past three generations. My grandparents worked a small farm, yet

I continue to kill even the most hardy of houseplants. I navigate with street signs and Mapquest, not from any innate knowing which way is west by the sky. I grew up learning to think, not to feel my way through my environment. Others grew up differently. Lost in an urban environment, they thrive backpacking in the hills far away from any Internet connection. According to the Earth Institute at Columbia University, soon more of the earth's population will live in urban centers than rural areas. What could that mean for an individual human being's relationship to, and even thinking about, the planet? And what does that relationship have to do with deep writing?

If you are able, lie down on the ground. If you're not comfortable doing that, sit in your chair with your feet squarely on the ground. Whatever position works for you, begin to think consciously about what you're touching. Sure, first perhaps carpet or tile, then underneath that is the concrete flooring, then maybe there are levels of apartments underneath you, and then more cement and plumbing and pipes, but eventually, all roads lead to the earth. When we lie on or touch the ground, we recognize the strength and stability that comes from her. We are held up by her, supported by her, and even when she shifts, explodes, or floods, she's still there. And if she weren't—well, we all know the answer to that. We're not simply standing on our own feet. Those feet stand on something, which rests on something, which rests on something, which, ultimately, rests on the earth. More interdependency at work. When we write, we may feel like we're in isolation. Indeed, writing is often called the "solitary profession." But we're not alone. We're not working in a vacuum. Pay attention to how you stand. How you walk. How you move your body through your environment. How conscious are you of what you're doing?

Every week on *A Prairie Home Companion,* Garrison Keillor takes us back to Lake Wobegon. In January, when the weather in Phoenix is just becoming nice enough to go outside without a gallon of water, Garrison is talking about short gray days and blizzards and frozen pipes. I would look out my window in Phoenix at the cloudless sky, note the seventy-six-degree temperature and my sockless feet, and be transported to a place experiencing a condition I had never really encountered: winter. Through Keillor's weekly monologues, I become a Norwegian Lutheran or someone who makes Jell-O casseroles with marshmallows, or, shiver at the thought, an ice fisherman. I recently read Jonathan Lethem's novel *Fortress of Solitude.* Through that breathtaking experience, I became a young boy growing up in Brooklyn during the 1970s. Lethem grew up in Brooklyn, and the place marked him, as our places mark all of us. His place became his source for that novel. Keillor uses Minnesota, his place, as the source for his work. In Phoenix, we talk about heat indexes and the number of days without rain. In Minnesota, they talk about snow and the number of days without sun.

What does your piece of the earth talk about? What stories are hidden in the houses? The unpaved streets? The rusted mailboxes? You don't have to travel the world to find your landscape. You've grown up in one, and whether you connect with it or know without a doubt you're in the wrong place, you're still affected by it. You know the tide schedules if you grew up on the coast. You pay attention to storm warnings. Tornadoes may be a part of your landscape. In Phoenix, the first hundred-degree day, usually in early May, begins the descent into summer. Most of the rest of the country emerges in summer. In Phoenix, we go under. We're all people. It's the place we're living in that shapes our behavior, attitudes, desires, and activities.

Every place has a language of its own. The language does not reside just in the dialect or colloquialisms of an area. The language is in the names of everyday items—is it pop or soda? Is it the TV, box, or tube? Are you taking the train, the underground, or the subway? Places give you vocabulary that your characters will use to communicate with each other. The who, the what, the where is the surface portion. But what about the underneath layer? What about the earth *under* the earth?

As writers, we are listeners. We listen not just to people, but to other living things—trees, rivers, ravens. We watch the interactions of all these things and how the web is woven by all the players. Over time we see that this character simply could not *be* in Maine or Newfoundland or South Africa. This character can only have come from Portland or New Orleans. You'll begin to know these things instinctively. When a character isn't working for you, one of the first questions to ask is, "What would happen if I moved her to a different place?" Then, you'll begin to attune yourself with the whispers of the earth underneath our man-made structures. What is the land beneath Manhattan saying? What is the secret language of the earth's core?

One of the best ways to illustrate the unique whispering of various places is in the context of storms. Storms occur everywhere, but different types of storms frequent different parts of the planet. Arizona is unlikely to see a tsunami. However, our dust storms can result in zero visibility. Think about the different places you've seen. How many places have you been where you've witnessed storms? How does a thunderstorm behave in North Carolina? Or a monsoon in the desert southwest? What does the land smell like after the storm? Is the rain soft and consistent or is it hard, fast, and gone? How do you think weather patterns affect the people? We name the really big storms. What if we named them all? What name would you give the noontime washing in Vancouver? The microburst in Texas? The long summer rain in Virginia? The flash flooding in Massachusetts?

Since moving to Prescott, I have noticed wind. In Phoenix, there was never any wind unless there was a storm, and then it was the serious telephone-pole-uprooting kind of wind. Prescott has wind every day. My wind chimes actually make sounds. I am watching *myself* change because I have changed the place I'm in. How often is the sun out? Is the weather counted in how many days in a row it hasn't rained or how many days in a row it has? These things shape your stories because they shape your characters. If your characters are in Seattle, don't describe the weather as if they're in Tucson. The folks in Seattle will know.

But what about those inner whisperings of the earth? Sometimes, it's easier to hear them if you take a trip outside of your regular climate zone. In Oregon, I was thrown back into a beginner's mind. I saw the world anew. I found myself faced with a constant question: "What is that?" I didn't know the trees, the flowers, the insects. I didn't know the angle of the sun as it set or rose. I didn't know how dark the night could be outside of a city. And for the few weeks I was there, I felt the earth breathing herself back into me. And I was shocked that I had somehow *missed missing* her.

As the Toni Morrison quotation says at the beginning of the chapter, "all water has a perfect memory and is forever trying to get back to where it was." So it is, I think, for your lives as writers. We wear the skins of our characters, who take us where they need to go. Then we shed the skins of the characters so new characters and voices can come. If we hold on too tightly to the characters we've come to love, we'll clog up the flow and prevent the next novel from coming in. Our characters will take us to their piece of earth so we can listen to it breathe. My mentor in graduate school, Alma Luz Villa-nueva, followed her characters from California to Santa Fe. Alice Walker, in *In Search of Our Mother's Gardens,* writes about Celie, her protagonist from *The Color Purple,* moving her from the south to northern California so she could tell Alice her story. My character, Zöe, in my novel *Bone Dance,* moved me from Phoenix to Prescott, AZ, and the characters who visit me here would not have shown themselves to me in Phoenix.

Our planet, our Earth, has seen billions of years of changes. Her core, hot and fiery, keeps us rooted to her. The earth, like our bodies, holds the stories of her growth and evolution. Drive the stretch of interstate between Albuquerque and Santa Fe. Underneath the billboards and casinos and convenience stores are ancient stories. You can walk through the Colliseum in Rome, surrounded by trendy boutiques and scooters and still hear the gladiators. Walk down the main street in your town and listen. Who or what do you hear? Listen *underneath* the first layer of sound—the people chatting, cars driving by, buses, music. Be still and listen deeper. What is the earth re-membering? Write it down.

Touchstones

1. Where are your roots? Describe the place any way you see fit.

2. Conjure a smell that reminds you of a place that has sig-nificance for you. Once you identify the smell, bring it fully into your body. Feel it around you. On your skin. In your throat. Now, drift to images. Don't try to control the im-ages. Let whatever surfaces be perfect. When you feel ready, begin to write. Let that smell be your entry point into the world.

3. Trees are a wonderful manifestation of rootedness and reaching, stability and stretching. By reaching down and up simultaneously, they open their centers, their hearts. The reaching *and* rootedness make "tree." Write your story through the history of your relationship with trees, or through a relationship with a particular tree.

4. Describe your relationship with the earth. Freewrite as long as it takes to get to the truth. When you get there, solidify that idea with a specific image. Then, on a separate piece of paper, begin a story, poem, or monologue with that specific image as the starting point.

13

INNER AND OUTER WORLDS

When we inhale, the air comes into the inner world.
When we exhale, the air goes out to the outer world.
The inner world is limitless, and the outer world is also
limitless. We say "inner world" or "outer world" but
actually, there is just one whole world.

SHUNRYU SUZUKI

ONE OF THE WAYS TO CREATE conflict in characterization
is to put the character's external actions and behaviors at odds
with the character's internal thoughts and feelings. This con-
trast gives the reader a broad insight into the character and
helps create tension in the narrative. Even if the inner and
outer worlds of your characters appear to be at odds with one
another, once you delve into the deeper mythology of your
characters you'll discover how the disconnects occurred and
why there is this chasm between them. It's important that you,
the author, know the how and why. Readers may not know
until the end of the book, if at all.

Sometimes we put on acts to go in public—we dress like

the lawyers we are when we'd rather be in sweatpants; we carry our portable electronics and respond to beeps and pages in a three-piece suit when we'd rather be camping in Yosemite. Have you ever put on a smile for your boss that you didn't truly feel inside? Told your great-aunt Sue, without truly meaning it, how lovely the chartreuse sweater with the pom-pom hat she gave you for your birthday was? How do you hide or bring forth what's inside?

Oftentimes, novels are about characters realizing their external and internal worlds don't mesh. If you, as the author, only consider the external traits, your characters will be flat. If you don't understand how the internal world is affecting the external world, your characters will be unbelievable.

Body Break

Hum! Take a deep breath in and exhale with sound through closed lips. Experiment with different tones and intensities with your humming.

Why? Sound helps rouse the brain, throat, and cells. It helps us listen with our inner ear. As the sound vibrates through our bodies, our internal organs are touched, awakened, and stimulated. We wake up from the inside out.

John Gardner's term "fictive dream" is one of the most accurate terms for describing the experience you are giving your reader. You're providing a place for her to fall into, just as sleep does for dreaming. A place where she can surrender the dream of her life and fold into the dream of the story. You cast the spell, and she is compelled to stay with the magic of your story, at least until the end of the book. Disruptions in the fictive dream are like continuity gaffes in films. The reader is pulled out of the dream, suddenly, if she is confused by a phrase or a character, or by factual inaccuracies or continuity issues. Or, if she can't connect with the characters because they are too paper thin to have substance, or they are too sloppily drawn to be clear.

When we have a recognizable form (an outer image, or outer line) filled in with gorgeous splashes of color, we have a painting that commands attention. It is the same with both the characters in your work and the work itself. A novel or poem has an outer line, a container, that is solid, holding the threads of story and language together inside. This container is our craft—the way we use structure, language, and imagery to anchor the reader. We build that outer edge so people will know how to carry our work. So they'll know how much it weighs and where to keep it. Without this line, this structure, this shape, readers don't know how to approach a work. Our left brain needs to classify, categorize, and identify something before it lets us surrender to it. Is it poetry? A novel? A how-to book? The package, the form, helps us find the doorway in.

A solid structure helps the reader enter the dream. But, you can't attach to the structure too much in the prewriting stage. Think about it like choosing luggage pieces before you know where you're traveling. If you use an overnight bag for a six-week trip to Asia, you've got the wrong bag. Likewise, a steamer trunk is probably a bit much for a weekend trip with friends. But of course, we have to start somewhere. As we figure out what we need to pack (Do you really need three pair of nearly identical black shoes or is one pair enough? Did you pack the essentials—underwear, toothbrush, soap?), we'll find, or, more accurately, the contents will dictate, the right suitcase for the trip. Start from the inside and work to the outer edge. Then, when you figure out what really needs to go on the trip with you, take away everything else. No sense carrying extra weight (needless words) out into the world.

Flat, undeveloped characters, stories, and poems occur when there is not an organic relationship between the lines themselves and what's inside them. One or the other is forced, superimposed, or not defined enough to form an organic union with the other part. When we start out writing, we chip at the surface of what it can be. Some places seem impenetrable, while others dissolve underneath us, revealing the layer that was holding it up. It's like an oval. At the top, we start where the energy feels most compelling. As we move deeper, we descend in a spiral, uncovering more and more until we find the core of our piece. Then, we begin moving up in a narrowing spiral, discarding the elements that don't fit this particular project.

When we break ground again, we're carrying to the surface only that which is necessary, but *knowing* that we could not have known what was necessary if we hadn't uncovered all we could. The most precise decisions come from the widest array of choices. Give yourself those choices, so you can give the reader the substance she's craving. When there is union between the outer and inner worlds of your work, then the boundary or veil between them dissolves and the reader enters *your* dream, takes her sustenance from it, and merges back into *her* dream, taking with her the things that mattered most from the experience.

Touchstones

1. This exercise is called "inside out." Take a piece you've written and identify the heart of it. Ask yourself if the structure (outer line) fits the content. Does the content fit within the structure? Where have you underpacked? Overpacked? Revise accordingly.

2. Reread a book or poem you found captivating. This time, read with the eyes of a writer. Take notes on areas where you can see the craft choices the author made to create the fictive dream. Can you illustrate the structure (outer line)? What were the things that filled in the spaces? Be specific. Don't just say "plot" or "setting." Find specific lines and phrases that worked. How, specifically, did the author weave the fictive dream? Don't say, "She's a good writer." *How* is she a good writer? *What* choices did she make and *why* do you think she made them?

14

SHADOW BOXING

The gift turned inward, unable to be given, becomes
a heavy burden, even sometimes a kind of poison. It
is as though the flow of life were backed up.

MAY SARTON

DEEP WRITING IS more than just communication with
others. It is, at its center, a conversation with the self. I know
more about my students than they think they're revealing to
me, not because I'm that brilliant and astute, but because their
inner lives are laid out on the page, most of the time without
their knowledge. Reading authentic creative work reveals the
author's persistent questions. It reveals what is still not under-
stood, what is still simmering, what is unresolved. The plot
in the writing could be taking place on a spaceship, but the
authenticity of the themes belies the humanity of the author.

The heartbeat of truth beats beneath every fictional story.
Rather than run from this, embrace it. It's part of the mystery
of what you're doing. As you grow as a writer, you'll build up
files of work. Take a trip back from time to time and reread
older pieces. You'll see things in the work you'd have never
imagined at the time you wrote it. You'll see, if you journeyed

to your center, your deepest self speaking to you through the work. As you observe this, you'll begin to trust that your writing is more than just the "thinking you" sitting at the desk. You'll see that it is helping you work with things that are troubling you, whether it's something gigantic like global warming or something more personal like your relationship with your brother. The type of writing and the kind of processes I'm showing you in this book are designed to help you communicate more effectively with that part of yourself that you may not be aware exists. Sounds impossible. But really, it's not only quite possible, it's necessary. Through writing you bring more and more things that have been hidden to the surface. You bring the darkness into the light over and over and over again.

Every human being has a shadow side. This shadow side contains ideas, feelings, desires, that he believes are not "good" or appropriate to bring to the public. Things in the shadow are not evil, though, they are simply hidden from view. A child who grew up in a family that did not allow her to speak her mind might have hidden her authentic voice away so she could survive within the confines of her childhood home. A child who was taught that being a man meant being aggressive might hide his gentleness in the shadow part of his psyche. Quite often, as Carl Jung tells us, what is in the shadow is "pure gold." Through acculturation, we tend to hide those very qualities that would sustain us. We may push our drive to write down deep because it isn't practical, and we find ourselves accountants. We hide our tremendous capacity for compassion because we got hurt once and decided it's safer not to be loving.

Our shadows are half of ourselves. We don't want the shadow side to disappear. If it does, we will be flat. Nor do we want the shadow to take over our psyches. This is another way the sun and moon qualities (light and dark, yang and yin) are represented in our bodies. We are looking for integration, not dissolution of one and dominance of the other. The tricky thing about our shadows is that we don't usually have much of an idea of what is in there. Have you ever wondered where a mean comment that just seemed to fall out of your mouth came from? Have you ever found yourself irritated at someone for no reason you can identify? Have you ever done something "out of character" that surprised you and others? Any of these situations, and many more, are calling cards from your shadow.

Psychologist James Hillman says,

> The unconscious cannot be conscious; the moon has its dark side, the sun goes down and cannot shine everywhere at once, and even God has two hands. Attention and focus require some things to be out of the field of vision, to remain in the dark. One cannot look both ways.

Currently, many people's outlooks are dualistic. There is a clear right and wrong, a good and evil. You are either with us or against us. Dualistic thinking won't lead you into deep writing or deep living. Dualistic thinking divides and allows us to falsely believe that we are chosen while they (whoever the "they" of the moment are) are damned. This dualism results in a society that attempts to banish everything it deems unacceptable, and it devotes a great deal of time and energy to banishment. Remember, when we attack, we feed that very thing we are hoping to destroy. We give power precisely to those characteristics we wish to see disappear when we invest our precious energy into the "fight." Don't engage in pursuing outward enemies; instead, strive to understand the conflicting energies inside yourself.

Writing is one way of doing this work. But it's warrior work. We don't want to see the selfishness inside us. We don't want to acknowledge that, given a different context, we might have been a terrorist or a murderer or a thief. We don't want to say to someone who we think has done the unforgivable, "Yes, I can see a part of me in you." But until we can do that, we can't access the deepest potential of ourselves as artists and human beings. We don't have to become a criminal to recognize that underneath the *behavior* is a motivation for love, connection, or acceptance that we can relate to. Shadow work shows us that we are much more than the whitewashed versions we put on the block for public viewing. Shadow work wakes us up to the depth of the human animal. Jung said,

> The individual who wishes to have an answer to the problem of evil has need, first and foremost, of self-knowledge that is the utmost possible knowledge of his own wholeness. He must know relentlessly how much good he can do, and what crimes he is capable of, and must beware of regarding the one as real and the other as illusion. Both are elements within his nature, and both are bound to come to light in him, should he wish—as he ought—to live without self-deception or self-delusion.

What doesn't fit in our idealized self falls into the shadow. It's what happens when we live in a culture. Some qualities are praised while others are shamed. We adapt accordingly so we can find acceptance.

When I talk about the shadow, it's important to understand that I'm talking in metaphors. We can't walk into a store and buy a shadow self. Nor can I go home, look deeply into a mirror, and see a dark figure lurking behind my eyes. I see manifestations of it in my behavior and the behavior of others. Great literature often explores the shadow. Some of our favorite characters, such as Dr. Jekyll and Mr. Hyde and the Phantom of the Opera, are metaphors for our shadow selves. We can look at the story of *Phantom of the Opera* literally. A young woman mourns the death of her father. She has a great singing talent, but falls in love and is abandoning her talent to pursue the excitement of romance. A mysterious phantom living in the theater begins to haunt her, ultimately capturing her and trying to possess her. We can take the Phantom character as a literal character, or we can look at the Phantom's character as a manifestation and metaphor for Christine's muse. As she represses or ignores her singing talents, her muse gets louder. Christine's gift was her voice. When she chose to be with Raul instead of committing herself to her music, the Phantom got jealous. If we look at the Phantom not as a wounded man, but as a part of her psyche, it changes the whole story.

In addition to individual shadows, there are cultural shadows. The cultural shadow is the larger framework within which the individual shadow develops. There are things that a particular culture may discourage or encourage that are completely the opposite in other cultures. For example, Americans value independence and individualism, whereas other cultures consider community and sharing of resources to be more important. Again, there is no "right" or "wrong"; there are only the storylines we have accrued in a lifetime that create the "I" that we use to navigate the world. Our awareness of our own storylines is essential to deep writing.

One easy way to see some of the things in our own shadows is to look at our projections. What ideas and qualities do we project onto an individual or a situation? Here are two examples of projection from my life, one toward an object and one toward an individual.

I taught a weekend writing workshop in Tucson several years ago. I got into town late, had trouble falling asleep because there was a wedding going on in the courtyard of my hotel, and overslept. I was told there would be some food in the morning at the workshop location, so I skipped breakfast in order to get to the classroom on time. I didn't tell the person in charge of the food table what I wanted for breakfast; I had just assumed there would be something I would like. However, since I didn't ask for what I wanted, the table didn't have what I needed. When the food I desired wasn't there, I was grumpy. The breakfast table became inadequate, bad, almost evil because I was projecting my dissatisfaction onto the table. The table itself was just neutral. It was simply a table with food on it. My story, my projections, my desires, created my judgment of it.

This next example is more personal. A few years ago, I found myself angry with my friend who had just broken up with an ex-lover of mine. She had moved on and was excited about the potential of her new relationship. I noticed I was getting angry at her for not staying with my ex. Because I knew something else was going on, I was aware enough not to express the anger at her. I began to journal about my feelings toward my friend, and what I found at the root of it was that I was still carrying anger toward my mother for remarrying after my dad's death. My anger had nothing to do with this woman, my ex, or her new relationship. It was my shadow self projecting my unacknowledged feelings onto a target that closely represented parts of the situation I still had not resolved. This awareness I gained prevented me from acting out toward her or my ex. It prevented me from acting out with my mother, and it showed me where I still have some work to do around my family dynamic. It was a gift. Had I not acknowledged that I was angry at all, these feelings would have continued to go underground, perhaps manifesting in a way that was harmful to my relationships or myself. We can't be too careful when it comes to our shadow selves. The more intimate our relationship is with it, the more quickly we recognize its signals and integrate its messages without causing harm to people we care for.

The shadow contains a wealth of knowledge about ourselves. As writers, we're seeking to live without self-deception or self-delusion. We're seeking a way through the mysteries of the world. We're seeking to make meaning from the chaos we see all around us. Don't be afraid of or oppose that which is within your own flesh. Awareness allows you to work with it without causing harm to yourself or others. Awareness opens; fear closes. When in doubt, choose opening.

Touchstones

1. Triggers are behaviors or actions that have a tendency to set you off in some way. Do you know what your triggers are? Make a list of them. Write a scenario in which you are triggered. For example, if you have a tendency to pick up a beer when you feel attacked at the office, write out that scene. Include the person you feel is doing the attacking and you, as yourself, responding to the attack. Be honest. After you have written this scene, rewrite the scene in which you make a different choice. How is the outcome different? Read the new scene aloud. What do you feel when you read it? If you feel tightness or an emotion surfacing, *allow it to be with you.* Do not try to push it away. Do not try to ignore it or shift the focus of your work. Just allow it to be. Breathe into it, keeping both feet grounded on the floor.

2. Freewrite: "If no one would object, I would . . ." Follow this with: "If no one would object, I would stop . . ."

3. What do you passionately desire from your creative work? When do you feel most alive and inspired? What is the stone that you push uphill, that is, the burden that opposes and resists you in this work? What shadow character sabotages your efforts in this work?

4. What is the emotion you are least in touch with? Draw it. Dialogue with it: Who are you? Where do you live? What do you want? What will happen if I access you? Why have you been so quiet? What do you have to tell me?

5. What themes emerge in your own work? Which one is most compelling to you now? Dialogue with it: Why do I care about you so much? How can exploring you help me? How can it help others? If you could tell me one thing that would help me on my journey with you, what would it be? Write a poem/prose piece around the theme.

15

OBSERVATION

The mind which yields to the wandering senses
carries away his wisdom as a gale carries away a
ship on waters.

BHAGAVAD GITA 11:67

IT SHOULD COME AS NO SURPRISE to anyone who has tried to sit down and write more than an e-mail that writing requires great mental discipline. Our fast-paced, media-focused culture has made it harder and harder for us to cultivate the mental discipline necessary to deepen our lives. We have hundreds of cable channels to choose from, sound bytes of news on the Internet, podcasts, and schedules that are impossible to maintain. Everything around us, from the billboards on the freeways and buses to the constant drone of television that provides the soundtrack to many people's lives, bombards us with sensory input. It is extremely hard not to get distracted from the task at hand, whether it be writing a book or playing with your child.

We have to make a conscious choice to withdraw from this daily assault on our senses. Our bodies and minds are highly adaptable; they filter everything around us, and we construct our lives through this filtering. We experience the world not as it is, but as our nervous system responds to it. Think about that for a minute. We are set up, as humans, to filter the world around us so we can function. If we could see, hear, smell, taste, and touch everything within our reach, we would become paralyzed.

Mother Teresa said, "If there are a hundred children hungry, and you can feed only one, feed one. Don't worry about the ninety-nine you can't feed. If you did, you'd end up doing nothing. And do it today. Tomorrow the child will be dead." Think about this quotation in the context of your writing. Can you possibly write down everything you experience? Can you write *all* the novels in you to write? All the poems? Many students freeze when confronted with the stunning amount of work they are *capable* of doing. Don't freeze. Focus. Select an object of attention and stay with it.

The practice of withdrawing your senses can be very beneficial to writers. Sense withdrawal helps us to focus more keenly on what is important. It gives us the space to move deeper into our stories and attempts to connect us with ourselves.

I was in Phoenix visiting an old friend recently when we decided to go out to dinner. He lives in a very trendy part of town, and we both knew what going out would mean—lots of people, lots of chatter, lots of sensory input. Almost every restaurant near him, including the fast-food options, has a television in it. Most have a series of televisions in each room, and some even have televisions in the floor. My friend mentioned getting a pair of glasses with dark arms to block out the pull of the televisions so he could focus on whom he was with. Television is a common example of how we get pulled out of where we are on a daily basis. As my friend and I ate dinner, our gazes wandered from time to time to the images on the screen, whether it was the March Madness scores or the weather update. We were aware of this and had to laugh, but we both knew it was really no laughing matter.

How can we pay attention to our lives—our real lives, not the outward trappings that are often labeled as life—if we have distractions at every turn? Our minds provide a lifetime of distractions to work with. When we combine our own natures with the sensory overload most of us live with every day, we have more than enough work to do just trying to hear our own voices—something essential for every writer.

Body Break

Place your index finger and middle finger of your right hand on your left wrist until you feel the beating of your heart. If you are having difficulty locating your pulse, place your fingers on the side of your neck. If you are still having difficulty finding your pulse, place your right hand directly over your heart.

Why? This will help pull you back into the body and ground you into your own internal rhythm. By focusing on the beating pulse, you will begin cultivating observation and listening skills without judgment.

A writer's voice is nothing deep and mysterious. Voice can be tricky to define because it manifests differently in different people, but it is not something amorphous and present only in "great" writers. Writers struggle to find their voices because they struggle with the process of listening. When we as writers talk about finding our voices, we mean: What do I sound like when there is nothing and no one else speaking? What do I have to say once the distractions of my life are stilled? It takes a bit of travel on the writer's path to learn how to be still—not just physically, but mentally—long enough to hear what he sounds like.

The instinct of many a novice writer to "go away" from his current life to find his voice is, I think, largely correct. However, this path is often unsuccessful because the writer doesn't understand the reason he can't hear himself speak is not because he lives in New York or Wichita, but because he hasn't learned how to withdraw himself from the world around him and simply listen. Paris will be *different* from home. A writing retreat in coastal Oregon will be *different* from home. But both will still contain whatever distractions the writer carries with him to stay disconnected from himself.

How can detaching from the senses help a writer? I know it sounds crazy. Haven't we been told, since writing our very first descriptive paragraph in fourth grade, to be specific? Use sensory language! What did that ocean smell like? How did the breeze feel on your face? All these questions come up in any writing class. And rightfully so. We do need solid, concrete details in order to connect with the story. Without specifics, the reader and the story flounder. So why would it be helpful to withdraw from this vital part of writing?

First, we're not *eliminating* the senses. Withdrawal from is not the same as negating. We're not talking about the absence of sensory input, but rather how to work with a precision of input. Second, sensory withdrawal helps us learn to focus more intently and completely on the object of our attention (our plot conflict, our character's crisis moment, our description of the wedding scene).

For example, I've been paying attention to my own mental tendencies as I've been writing this chapter. The buzzer on the clothes dryer has gone off several times. I've responded with relief. Ah! I get to move, stretch, and take care of the things of the world, like clean clothing. I've poured and drunk three cups of coffee, eaten more than a handful of M&M's, and watched the fish swim in the fish tank. After writing for about a half an hour today, I looked out my window and noticed it was snowing. Since learning it was snowing outside, I've stopped after almost every sentence to look outside and see if it was still snowing. While I'm gazing outside, I think about how that snow will affect my plans for tomorrow. I wonder how much will fall. Last weekend we had over a foot. Will it be more than that? Less? Then I think about the drought. Arizona is currently in a seven-year drought. Is this snowfall going to help? Is it too little too late? Then I think about the urban sprawl in Phoenix. Where is the water coming from for all those people? What will happen if we really don't get enough rain? And then, at last, I feel the pen in my hand again and I remember I'm writing now. I need to pull inward so I can hear what I want to say. I need to withdraw from the sensory input around me so I can focus on what I'm doing. Right here. Right now. Oh yes.

Think about all the things you observe on any given day. Because of the sensory onslaught most of us live with, we filter the input in order to function. How do you discern what to let in and what to filter out? How do you determine what is meaningful (the sudden drop in barometric pressure) with what is insignificant (the bus was five minutes late)? This is a writing question too. Which details matter and which ones are filler? The answers lie with the story. A drop in barometric pressure or a late bus can be important or unimportant. Each answer creates a different story.

My cat practices sensory withdrawal every time she sees a bird outside the window. When a raven catches her eye, she leaps from whatever she's doing and makes a mad dash for the window, where she stiffens, focuses on the black bird, and begins the clack-clacking of her tongue designed to lure the bird to her. I can clap my hands next to her ears and she won't move. I have even picked her up and carried her away from the window, but her gaze never leaves the bird, and as soon as I release her, she's back in the window, focused, taunting the object of her attention. She achieves this focus by withdrawing from her surroundings so she can attend to the job at hand— chasing the bird. If she responded to every bit of stimuli in the house, she would never be able to see the bird, let alone try to catch it.

Sensory withdrawal helps us deepen the experience of one small thing—the taste of the apple fresh from the tree, the smell of the season's first dogwood bloom, the texture of the skin on the second knuckle of our middle fingers. A good story or poem is made up of clear, specific images. The key writing piece in sense withdrawal is to learn to move from "every" thing to "one" thing. Don't tell us about how loving your grandmother was by using words like "love," "kind," and "special." Show us that experience by moving from the universal (love) to the specific. Start describing the cookie jar on the avocado green countertop. Is it shaped like Cookie Monster? A big chocolate chip cookie? Is it handmade by one of her grandchildren? Is it glass? Ceramic? A metal tin, perhaps? Can you remember a time when the cookie jar figured prominently in a family situation? The reader doesn't have to have had a cookie jar that looked just like the one you're describing to be able to make a personal connection to the *meaning* of that cookie jar. Your specific image created a specific image for them, which they can easily connect to the world at large. This connection is part of the magic of the relationship between the reader and the work. By practicing withdrawal of the senses, you will create a precision in your writing. You will gain clarity and focus. You will create a concrete image for the reader to connect with. You will learn to separate, pinpoint, and then elaborate.

Georgia O'Keeffe said, "There is nothing less real than realism. Details are confusing. It is only by selection, by elimination, by emphasis that we get at the real meaning of things." I picked up the postcard with this quote on it at the Georgia O'Keeffe Museum in Santa Fe one summer. I had always been intrigued by O'Keeffe's work; her broad strokes and seemingly simple style created deep impressions in me. I picked up the postcard initially because I was troubled by the quote. I didn't understand it. It sounded like a Zen koan. How could realism not be real? What is realism anyway? Her paintings—the essence of a tree in winter, the opening of a calla flower, the brilliant white of a cow's skull—provoked such intense feeling in me. For me, they were more powerful than the paintings of other artists who strove to capture every single leaf on every tree in the forest. I thought about what has been traditionally considered "good" art. If the artist can successfully copy the world around her, does that make the art "good"? If she is able to select and emphasize a single defining image of the world around her, is that somehow better?

I didn't have the answers to these questions, but I began looking at my students' writing and my own through the lens of sensory withdrawal. How many details are there? How long do we really have to describe the rock before the reader can see it too? How muddled is the language when details become cumbersome? Where do I get confused as a reader? Where do I disconnect from the story because I feel like the author is demanding I see the world the exact same way he does?

I noticed that the more the author "told" me, the less I connected to the story. Likewise, when an author created sensory overload in a scene, trying to "show" me too much, I could no longer see, hear, smell, taste, or touch any part of the story. Yet, when the author practiced restraint and gave me only key bits of each scene, I found I was able to move much more deeply into the characters and the conflict. I was able to participate more fully in the scene because of simply that: I was allowed to participate in the scene. Everything wasn't handed to me. I could make my own interpretations, with the author's guidance and anchoring in the things he felt were critical to show me.

The reader wants to participate in the characters' lives too, not just be a receptor for the author's information and agenda. How do we know what is important to give the reader? We practice. And we learn that every story requires different techniques. We also learn to distinguish between the *significant* details and the details that clutter. Sensory withdrawal helps us do this. As O'Keeffe says, "It is only by selection, by elimination, by emphasis that we get at the real meaning of things."

Let's practice.

Touchstones

1. Let's begin with the body. Lie on your back, arms by your sides, palms up. Let your feet fall naturally to the sides. As you lie on the floor, draw your attention to your toes and feel the warmth in them. Then, move your attention to your ankles. Then to your knees, your thighs, your belly, your heart. Then, begin again with your fingers, moving to your wrists, your elbows, your shoulders, your throat. Then, draw your attention to your jaw, releasing it. Then to your eyes and your third eye (the space between and just above your eyebrows). As you focus on each specific area of the body, let the rest of the world around you fade away. Think only of your toes, your knees, your belly. Then

release that focus as you move to the next part. You may lie on the floor as long as you choose to. Notice how the world drops away. When you are ready to sit up, begin to move slowly. Bring awareness back into your toes and fingers. Deepen your breath. Roll gently over to one side and push yourself up to a seated position. Observe which parts of the outside world return to you first. Pick up your journal and begin to freewrite. You might choose to focus on a particular body part, or you might try to capture the entire experience. You might choose to dive deeply into the initial re-awakening as you moved from lying down to sitting up.

2. Take your journal and go to a favorite place. Once you get settled, focus on one of the five senses. Freewrite for ten minutes just on what you can see. Then move to what you can hear. Follow with the senses of taste, touch, and smell. Observe what you have to leave out in order to focus intently on one sense. How does that affect your overall impressions of the scene? Observe what challenges came up as you tried to separate one sense from the other, e.g., how is the sense of touch affected by the sense of sight?

   When you finish writing on each of the five senses, write a description of the place incorporating all you've observed. How has your impression of the place shifted now that you've dived into deeper places?

3. Describe a full moon from the point of view of someone who cannot see.

4. Being aware of the connection between the senses, practice with these exercises: Describe the taste of broccoli; the smell of clothes fresh from the dryer; the smell of earth after a heavy rain; the taste of chocolate to someone who has never eaten it; describe a physical pain (don't say it

hurts!); describe a fight between a husband and a wife witnessed by someone who can't hear.

5. Now let's work with describing emotions with strong details. Try these: describe a feeling of aloneness. Don't use the words "alone," "lonely," etc. Use specific imagery to create that feeling; next, describe a feeling of joy. Don't use the words "happy," "joyful," etc.

6. Pull out a story, poem, or essay you've been working with. Find a place in the piece where you use description. Look at the passage using sensory withdrawal. Do you over-describe, thus slowing down the action too much? Do you underdescribe? Have you left out significant details that the reader needs to understand the scene? Rework the passage based on your findings.

16

FOCUSED AWARENESS AND IMAGERY

Cast off what doesn't serve you before it robs you of your life.

NECAHUAL

NECAHUAL, MY MAIN CHARACTER in my novel, *Bone Dance*, spoke those words while standing on the edge of the Rio Grande. I often find out much later how wise my characters are and how much they have to teach me. At first, this was just a cool line. But I began to integrate it into my writing life and bit by bit began to focus deeper, casting aside what did not pertain to what I needed at that moment. That line helped me learn to focus and move deeper into the truth of my story.

Through cultivating a focused awareness we can build concrete imagery. In the previous chapter, we honed our observation skills by moving from one sense to another. In this chapter, we'll stay put, really moving deeply into an object, to create the concrete writing we need to communicate effectively. A popular writing adage is: Through the specific, we become universal. Simply put, this means we don't write about love. We write instead about a specific time when we gave or received love. Through a specific story, with its unique sensory language, dialogue, and characters, the reader will connect to her own experience of love. The reader will be able to *make meaning* from the experience you've written about. Without this specific story, we wind up writing things like, "Love is great" or "Love sucks," depending on our current experience. How much more effective is it to slow down and deliver the richness of the *story*?

Readers respond to specific language. Vague or abstract terms can't be seen, so they can't be integrated and remembered. In order for us to write specifically, we need to learn how to slow down and move into the scene, rather than gloss over the scene in our hurry to either meet our output goal or avoid the real work of the scene.

Most of us face the second problem: avoiding the real work of the scene. Because writing stirs things up, uncovers things, brings us face to face with the unexpected, we can be sure that some discomfort will occur when we sit down to write. Rather than following our perfectly planned outline, our authentic self has something else in mind, and we find ourselves suddenly in uncharted waters. We end up uncomfortable, and without the tools to deal with this discomfort, we leave the work, skim over the critical moments of change in the story, or stop writing entirely.

I wish I had a dollar for every student's story or novel chapter I've read that summarized the climactic scene in two short sentences. It almost feels like an assault to the reader. Pages read, time invested in building interesting characters, setting up a strong situation, building tension only to find—WHAM!—the author hits and runs, leaving the reader holding unraveled storylines like pieces of old twine. Inevitably, this happens because the author couldn't hold the space for the scene to unfold. He couldn't be with the emotions moving through him. She couldn't sit with the inactivity of the character or step back outside of herself and the story to that place of witness consciousness to allow the story to take its own direction.

Releasing control is frightening. To leap off the abyss, we have to believe something will sustain us. Going deep into our authentic voice is very unsettling because it is often very unfamiliar. If we are not in the practice of speaking from and living from that authentic place, what will it sound like when it speaks? What will it reveal that we have been trying to hide? If we *react* to what comes up, it will most likely get us out of the chair and into some other activity that distracts us. If we give in to the chatter in our minds, we will be pulled from our work into something that momentarily gives us relief from whatever emotions were emerging from doing the work. But, like all distractions, it will only be a temporary fix. We will once again find ourselves having to choose between doing the work and doing something else. We may fight the writing. Or we may negotiate with it or attempt to ignore it. But sooner or later, we either write or we don't. And if we do, we must return to the chair.

The insidious part of the writing process is that it will continue to reveal to us where we need to go. The next time we sit down to write, once again, the unfamiliar authentic voice or idea or emotion will surface. Once again, we have the choice to stay and be with what comes up, focusing clearly on each feeling, each character, each blade of grass, each rumble of a car engine that moves through our story. Or, we move to the next distraction. Stories are layers that can only be uncovered by focusing long enough to see what's underneath. What we think we want to write about is just the visible surface of what is there for us to write about. As we approach that surface and crack it, we will find the hidden depth of our stories. We will find that lingering awhile in the unfamiliar parts of our writing brings us surprising twists and revelations about our work.

Consider the difference between riding in a car at sixty miles per hour along a small two-lane road in rural North Carolina compared to walking that same road at a leisurely pace. What additional things do you think you'd discover? What unexpected flowers might you see? What bird sounds might you hear? How many textures of earth, of fencing, or of trees might you be able to touch? What new paths might you take because you caught a glimpse of something interesting underneath a rock or deep in the woods?

Slowing down and focusing your awareness will help you stay in the moment of your writing so that you can follow those unanticipated paths into the forest. By focusing on what is presently in front of you, you cannot be concerned with the destination point. Releasing the outcome will release the work.

In 1999, I traveled to Italy with some friends. We stayed in Rome a few days. On one of the days, we decided to take a bus tour to Pompeii. I had spent eight years of my life studying Latin. In fifth grade, I did a class project on Mount Vesuvius, complete with volcano and red play dough lava, so I was eager to see the actual site. We caught the bus at dawn and rode southeast to Naples, then on to Pompeii. Pompeii is a very popular tourist attraction, even in December, and our tour guide had his routine down to a science. He spoke broken English in a loud voice. He made it very clear that we had three hours for the tour. The bus would not wait. If we got lost, stayed in the gift shop too long, or wandered off the path, we would be left behind.

At each point of interest along the way, he recited his paragraph or two about the bathhouse, about the orgies that would go on in the fields under the full moon, about the bodies instantly mummified mid-stride as the lava poured out of the volcano in A.D. 79. We were one of dozens of tour groups. The same spiel was going on in Japanese, French, German, Spanish, and Italian. I couldn't take it all in. I needed to stop for hours. I needed to sit in the bathhouse, run my fingers over the grass, try to memorize the facial features of the woman who died trying to shield her infant from the lava with her body. I needed to be with these things long enough to absorb them, to make a part of them mine so I could one day write about them.

But we were on a schedule. Buses wait for no woman, no matter how pure her intentions might be. When it was time to move to the next point of interest, our guide clapped his hands enthusiastically and exclaimed, "Take your time quickly!" The first time we heard it, my friends and I burst out laughing. Our guide did not find this amusing. "Take your time quickly" became our mantra throughout Italy. Trains barely slowed down at the platform long enough for us to leap on with our too-heavy American luggage. Take your time quickly. In four words, our guide had summed up American culture. On a three-hour tour of Pompeii bracketed on both sides by a three-hour bus ride to and from Rome, I experienced American culture in a way I had not realized in America.

When we take our time quickly, we don't experience focused awareness. When we take our time quickly with our writing, we find ourselves writing things like, "We traveled to Pompeii on a bus. We ate bad spaghetti as the "included" lunch fare of the tour. We saw artifacts and ruins and had the opportunity to buy genuine Italian rosary beads. We got back in the bus and arrived in Rome after midnight." There's no *story* in that. No texture. None of the details or imagery that would allow anyone else to go on that trip with me.

Jim Krusoe, one of my writing teachers in graduate school, gave a talk about writer's block. He claimed there was no such thing. Whenever you get stuck, he said, slow down and write five sentences about each sense in your scene. Write five sentences on what your character sees, five on what she hears, and so on. Do that and then you'll know where to go next in the story. I didn't really believe him, but I tried it the first time I got stuck. It worked. I tried it the second time and it worked. By the third time, I didn't need any more convincing. What he was telling us to do was to stick around long enough to let the scene speak. By lingering in the sensory component of the scene, we stay grounded. We focus on what makes the scene breathe—a scene's vitality comes from its earth—its cellular makeup.

The reader enters a scene through her senses. That means the author has to show up long enough to experience them herself. The author has to engage in focused awareness in order to stay there so he can bring his readers there.

In the physical body, we practice focused awareness by observing and not avoiding whatever sensations come up within the body. We practice mindfully staying with the sensations that occur—the ones that are painful and the ones that feel good. As we practice this and don't react physically by pulling out of the situation just because we are uncomfortable folding forward for two minutes, we learn instead something far more valuable: how the mind responds to discomfort. We notice that it often responds as if it were being burned alive whenever its demands are not met, *regardless* of the reality of the given situation. We notice that even though we have been in forward fold for two minutes and are not being tortured or attacked by wild animals, our mind moves to Red Alert status the moment we tell it, "No, I am staying here." It tries everything it can to convince us that we are indeed in mortal danger and we must move *now* or else we will surely *die* (melodrama intended). These same messages surface when we sit down to write. Almost as soon as we commit to the practice, our egos start chattering as loudly as necessary for us to abandon the journey.

Body Break

Choose any position you like that feels comfortable and safe to you. You can sit in a chair, lie on a bed, stand on one foot or anything in between. Here's the challenge: Set a timer and remain in that position for five minutes, moving as little as possible. Use your breath to anchor you and keep you steady in the pose.

Why? This activity will help you observe in your body how quickly the mind wants to move on to the next thing. Notice how, even though you got to pick the pose, and you are not in any physical danger, you still want to get out of it into something else. Notice how the body begins sending you signals to move. Don't judge; just notice.

Caution: Of course, if you experience physical pain, please move out of the pose you've chosen.

Part of the physical practice is also staying with the mind as it rants and raves. As we continue to calmly tell it no, we begin creating a new habit. We begin learning how to be with whatever comes up without moving out of it. As we learn to do this in our bodies, we learn how to do this in our writing lives. We learn to say, "Yes, I see you. I feel you. I acknowledge you and I am not going to try and change you. I am going to be with you as long as you are here, and I know you will pass and change. Then I will be with what comes next."

When we are not putting forth effort to try to change our experience, we actually have the space to experience it. By not trying to make something different from what it is, we begin to teach ourselves to be less judgmental of all our experiences. When we accept what is, we can receive the gifts of the moment without conditions.

In writing, the magic of our stories lies in the unexpected gifts of the moment, not in our finely tuned and orchestrated road map and speedy finish to the end. Writing is a process of discovery. We can't discover what we already know, or think we already know, is there.

With focused awareness, we can concentrate on what emerges in each moment of the writing process. We can stay with every nuance of the scene to find the truth, the authenticity underneath what we see superficially when we "take our time quickly." Stick around for a few breaths. The mystery will find you.

Touchstones

1. Go to the mirror and look into your own eyes. Notice the wrinkles around the edges. Notice the thickness or thinness of your lashes. What color are your eyes, *really*? What do you see, looking into them, that others don't? Focus now on one of the wrinkles. Allow your gaze to soften and connect with just that wrinkle. What does it remind you of? What does it say to you? Pick up your journal and write the story of that wrinkle.

2. Set a timer for fifteen minutes and consciously clasp your hands together. Notice what comes up. Do your palms

sweat? Are you anxious? At ease? What do you notice in the flesh of your hands? How does it feel to be touching your own skin without purpose or agenda, just with compassion? Sit with the anxiety or fidgeting that might come up. When the timer goes off, pick up your journal and write.

3. Choose an object or item from the natural world. It could be a rock, a shell, a flower, a blade of grass. Place it on the table in front of you. Soften your gaze. Touch the object, really taking the time to pay attention to its texture, its smell, its coloring. The object is the door into your writing. As you begin to merge deeper with that object, write whatever comes up. When you get stuck, return to the object, staying with sensory details as much as possible, and keep the writing flowing. Stay with the writing five minutes longer than when you would choose to stop.

4. Take a work in progress where you feel stuck and reread it. Circle or otherwise note areas that are of significant interest to you. You don't have to know why. Trust your intuition. Return to those circled sections and begin again, only this time disregard what you know comes in front of and/or behind that particular scene or line. Start writing, not from the original work, but from what comes to you immediately after reading the problematic line or paragraph. It's OK to overdescribe here. You can always cut later. One detail leads to another, which may provide the key to the next direction of the chapter or poem. Experience the flow that is possible from focused awareness.

17

CHARACTERIZATION
Deep Questioning

The most erroneous stories are those we think we know best—and therefore never scrutinize or question.

STEPHEN JAY GOULD

WHO POPULATES OUR STORIES AND POEMS? I've talked about how we listen to the earth for our characters and how we listen to the body. I've talked about the need to show up for the work. The discipline. The presence of mind. In truth, I don't know where characters come from. I don't know why some of them are successful and some of them are not. I don't know why someone finds herself compelled to write about someone of the opposite gender who lived in an area of the world in a time period she's never experienced. It's just the way of things.

The best piece of advice I can dispense about characterization is, as the Greeks said, "Know thyself." Authentic writing is first and foremost an inward journey. Please emphasize the word *journey*. You won't finish in this life. You'll continue to find out things about yourself and you'll hopefully continue to grow and deepen your connection to yourself as you live your life. There is no end to what is inside you to explore. I don't know where all that comes from either, but it's there.

Inner work is warrior work, too. We live in a society that encourages and rewards distractions from this inner journey. We are encouraged to focus on the outward manifestations of who we are. Women's magazines give lip service to "inner beauty" and then show models with unattainable bodies on the front covers. We face this dualism every day. Advertisers pitch ways for us to reinvent ourselves with new cars, clothes, and drugs. Many of our religions have us seeking outward for salvation. Writers, too, seek outward for their material in the form of lofty ideas and ideals. We create character sheets that focus on the superficial—eye color, hair color, favorite movie, scariest moment. We sketch an outside—a shell—and then wonder where to go to fill it. These shells are the flat characters moving around in your stories. They're half alive. Half present. And more often than not, this is a reflection on the author as well. I'm not trying to insult anyone. I just want to make clear the relationship between how well we know ourselves and how well we can know our characters. We can't go deeper on the page than we go off the page. Deep writing comes from deep living.

Cultural anthropologist Joseph Campbell brought to the public discourse the concept of individual and cultural mythologies. He created connections between the most disparate of cultures through their stories and worldviews. He showed us how a worldview, a storyline, makes a world. Sam Keen, in *The Power of Stories,* builds on this idea by discussing the levels of myth (meaning story, not untruth) each of us operates on. We have many different filters that our experiences travel through. We are products of what we've accepted as well as what we've rejected. We can't *not* see what we've seen, and so a lifetime shapes us. We have input from our families, our neighborhoods, our schools, our churches, and our governments, as well as our own experiences. We pick and choose what seems relevant to us at the time. As we grow, we discard what no longer works and replace it with something else. Your characters also go through this process of growth and change, and, if you pay attention, you'll see that many books are shaped on a character's challenging and shedding of an old belief system (mythology) in favor of a new one.

Most of our fundamental journeys are internal journeys. They may also include an external journey, but there is almost always an inward shift of some kind away from an old or toward a new storyline. Many a character's itch for change comes from a dissatisfaction with the current storyline of his life. So, as authors, we deal fundamentally with belief systems. We have to be comfortable in them. We have to realize we have them and we have to realize that no other human on the planet has the exact same mythology as we do. Jump headfirst into your characters' mythologies. What do they believe about love? Why? What do they believe about the earth? The cosmos? Gender roles? Family roles? Who or what is their god? Don't be afraid of these questions. Ask them of yourself first. You might be surprised at what you believe that you didn't think you did. You might find an uncomfortable prejudice or a judgment about a political group hanging out. You might find you understand some small part of that "other."

Find awareness.

Ah.

You're growing.

It takes a person willing to do deep self-exploration to build deep fictional characters. Your characters need the level of deep inner work you do for yourself. Assigning them an eye color doesn't give them an essence. Giving them a job doesn't give them a life. Some characters are deeply reflective and introspective. Some don't scratch the surface of their lives. Stories contain all types because humans contain all types. A novel in which everyone shared the same worldview wouldn't contain any conflict or tension—the keys to moving narrative along.

Don't be afraid. Open your heart and open your eyes. See what new worlds are within you.

Touchstones

1. Go out for a day dressed up like your character. Embody him or her. Think about movement. Posture. Gestures. Eye contact. Pay attention to how *you* are responded to by others when you're dressed as someone else.

2. Write a monologue from the point of view of one of your characters beginning with, "I believe . . ." Then, write a scene in which the character goes against something she previously claimed to believe in.

3. Write a monologue from the point of view of one of your characters beginning with, "I would never . . ." Then, write a scene in which the character has to do that thing. What has changed in the story or with your awareness of the characters as a result of this scene?

4. What would your character *never* buy? Take a stroll through a thrift store and see what strikes you. When you find the object, buy it and take it home with you. Place it in your writing area. Notice how it feels to have that object nearby. How is your character reacting to it? How are you reacting to it? What is so repulsive about that object to your character? Use that object in a scene you're working on.

18

POINT OF VIEW

I Am Not "I"

Every man takes the limits of his own field of vision for the limits of the world.

SCHOPENHAUER

AS YOU MAY HAVE HEARD in a creative writing class or textbook, point of view, often noted on manuscripts as POV, is the most complex and critical craft component you've got to work with, no matter your genre. That's actually true. Sorry. There's no way around it. To be a writer, you've got to come to grips with the woolly mammoth of point of view. And yes, this goes for poetry, too! Since writers of many different levels may be picking up this book, I want to give you a brief overview of the terminology for point of view so we're all on the same page before we move to the underbelly of it.

First, don't confuse point of view with opinion. It's an unfortunate word choice, but it's the one we have. In creative writing, point of view means the vantage point (character and distance or who and where) from which the work is being viewed. We can choose from the following three points of view or *persons*:

First person = I (singular) or we (plural)
I went to the movies.
Second person = you (singular and plural)
You get in your car and you see he left the remnants
  of his rum and coke on the front seat.
Third person = he/she/it (singular) or they
  (plural)
She hurried through the crowd at Penn Station,
  following a whiff of aftershave that reminded her
  of someone she thought she'd never see again.

In first person, the character is narrating the story. The "I" is *not* the author except in memoir or other forms of nonfiction. Second person is not commonly used, especially in longer works. It uses direct address (you go to the movies) to make the reader the character. Third person has a narrator telling the story. Even though that narrator may be showing you the thoughts of a single character, the narrator is *not* the actual character.

In the third-person choice, you get to play with one of our most prized tools: distance—both emotional distance and distance of time and space—and there are varying distances you can use. You can be perched on a telephone pole three miles from your main character or you can be right behind your character's eyes. These distances are reflected in the range from third-person limited (staying with one character's perceptions and thoughts) to the godlike, third-person omniscient (all knowing) choice of the epics.

John Gardner, in his classic *The Art of Fiction*, called this technique "psychic distance." How far away are you from the person/people whose thoughts you are conveying? From where is the camera's eye viewing the scene? Are we right behind the eyeballs, or are we perched on top of the tallest oak tree in the land? Distance determines scope and intimacy. Generally, point-of-view issues are ironed out in the revision stage. We swoop in and out depending on how we want to create tension, pacing, and intimacy.

The most common point-of-view choices we see in contemporary literature are first person and third person limited (often you'll see novels with numerous third-person-limited narrators broken apart by chapters). If you're new to writing, I recommend sticking with these choices for awhile until you get the hang of all that point of view can do. Sometimes I think about point of view like my word processing program. I only use a tenth of what the computer program can do, and every project I start teaches me something new about it, so don't feel like you have to "get it" right off the bat. Point of view is best experienced through your own writing and through reading with an eye for the point-of-view choices the author made.

As I mentioned earlier, a first-person narrator, except in memoir and autobiography, is not the author. This is true of poetry, too. We cannot assume an "I" in a work is the author's voice unless we're clearly told that. While it's true that elements of the author are found in all of her characters, you'll save yourself a lot of embarrassment in critique sessions if you learn early not to address the author with, "You know when you killed the rabid bat on page 2 . . ." Unless the author specifically told you she was writing a personal narrative, that kind of assumption is not just ignorant, it's rude and sloppy thinking. Please do check out one of the craft books I recommended for more insight into point of view. I've only scratched the surface here, but hopefully we have a common vocabulary now.

There are many factors that go into deciding which point of view to use in any given story. The majority of these concern the characters themselves and the different ways the story would be served by their unique qualities and personal perspectives. Let's take a look at where these characteristics might come from and how they might affect point-of-view choices. Perhaps you're already starting to see how POV builds on empathy, curiosity, acceptance, deep characterization, and the shadow. When students first begin writing, their characters are often two-dimensional carbon copies of the parts of themselves they are most comfortable with. It takes a long time to navigate the murky waters of point of view and here's the biggest reason why:

> The way you (and I) see the world is nothing more or nothing less than the way you (and I) see the world. There are six billion souls who see the world in their own way. You (and I) don't see the world as it is; we see the world within the framework of our senses, language, mythologies, experiences, and limitations.

No human can view the world completely objectively. We can try, but the effects of our background are deep, subtle, and tangled. We see what we expect to see. Others see something completely different within the same scene. This is because that same scene pushes different buttons in different people based on that individual's experiences. Not to know this about yourself and the people around you does a great disservice to the writing. You're not a bad person because your way of seeing the world is limited. You are a *person*. Work to expand your experiences and your awareness, with the humble knowledge that your lens is clouded in ways you have yet to even recognize. Practice acceptance now. You are human.

The second point-of-view challenge a writer faces is detachment:

> The writer's ego must dissolve so the character and/ or narrator can move in. The writer cannot impose her morality on her characters. She cannot have them only engage in activities she has participated in.

The third point-of-view challenge is a doozy:

> *The writer must visit her shadow.* She's got to understand and empathize with the motivations of her characters. Unless she wants a novel populated with sweet, conflict-avoiding, non-prejudiced people (which, as you might imagine, makes for a pretty boring story), she's got to find a way to connect with the part of her that does and thinks things she finds unacceptable. She has to find the part of her that understands (but doesn't have to condone) Hannibal Lector's misguided search for love in Clarice Starling or Humbert Humbert's quest for love in the child, Lolita.

Point of view requires not just mastery of technique, but compassion for yourself and your fellow humans. And then you, gentle writer, must fall in love with your characters even as you watch them suffer, struggle, and maybe even die. And yes, you get to watch them fall in love, triumph, laugh, and play. The wider and more expansive your life is, the wider and more expansive (and more believable!) your characters will be. You are not the center of the universe, and that is just as it should be. If it were all you, where would anyone else fit in? All of us view the world through a slanted lens, and so do your characters. Their own lenses are slanted differently from yours, yet this slanting is what makes that particular story or poem what it is. Change the point of view, and you change everything.

Think about a recent family gathering. You "know" what happened. So does your mother, your sister, your cousin. Each of you would tell the story of the event and their story would vary based on each person's internal mythologies and their *distance* (both physical and emotional) from the event. Within each family member's mind, she or he is telling the truth. Note that the event (the family reunion) is neutral. It is only the perceptions of the individual people that make meaning of the event and make the story. Remember: events and objects are neutral. People and characters are anything but neutral.

Deciding on point of view ultimately requires a multitude of choices, many of which are intuitive, all of which affect the work fundamentally. It's a fun thing to play with during revision. What would my story be if Jake were the narrator instead of Tana? What would happen if I used first instead of third person? What would happen if I backed up a little and told the story from the vantage point (distance) of the backyard? What if I moved in a little closer? Play with it. Don't get stuck with one point-of-view choice in your repertoire. And for goodness' sake, don't think you have to stick with the one you started with.

When I began *Bone Dance* it was not only in third-person omniscient, but all my characters had different names than the ones they ended up with. Ultimately, the novel is told in multiple first-person voices with a third-person objective voice interjecting in short chapters within the narrative. I had to admit, after thousands of words, that third-person omniscient wasn't giving me what I needed for the story. The story, as I grew to understand it, showed me which point of view was necessary to tell it. I had to trust the story, and I had to let go of my original idea.

When working with point of view, the options are really endless. Be flexible with yourself. Experiment with it. Don't force a particular point of view choice on your story. Be still and listen, but keep your pen ready!

Touchstones

1. Think of a traumatic situation, such as a car accident or a funeral. Describe the event in a series of first-person monologues from fifteen different participants/attendees. Give each character his or her own voice and interpretation of the events. Don't stop after three! Keep going. Stretch!

2. This exercise works with supporting characters. Write two monologues, one from each of the points of view of two of your supporting characters. For each monologue, examine the following questions: Who are you? What do you want? What's in your way? What are you willing to risk?

3. Take two to three pages of a scene you're working on and rewrite it from the point of view of a different character in the scene. If it's a scene with only one character, change from first person to third person, or third person to first person. What did you learn?

19

CHANGE

The universe is change; our life is what our thoughts make it.

MARCUS AURELIUS ANTONINUS

ONE SPRING AFTERNOON LAST SEMESTER I was working in my office at the college where I teach when I heard rain on the roof. This is a big event in Arizona in the middle of a seven-year drought. I had just been outside, though, and it was sunny, warm enough for shirtsleeves. Like many colleges, we have only a few windows scattered through our offices, so I went in search of one to see what was happening. Dark clouds. Heavy rain. Others had come out of their offices. We smelled moisture through the walls and were happy. Then, the rain turned to hail—the real hail: round, thick, golf balls. And within fifteen minutes, the hail had turned to snow. Within an hour, the sun was back out, and when I left to go home, I didn't need a jacket. Because I spent so much of my life in Phoenix where the weather shifts are miniscule, I am still awed by the moving, morphing clouds of my mountain town. I have realized, too, that the weather, if we choose to pay attention to it, guides us through the natural changes that occur in every facet of our lives. I realized that the weather and her moods are indicative of our own physiological shifts.

For me, living in Phoenix took me away from this internal subtlety. Every day *seemed* the same to me (although I know there were dew point changes and wind shifts). The longer I lived there, the more my awareness of my self disappeared. I became (to me) the same, day after day, like the way I perceived my exterior world. I know many people thrive in areas where the weather is predictable, but I am not one of them. When I moved north, I found my life expanding and shifting every day, just like the weather. I began to notice my body in a more intimate way. It, too, was different every day. Places that were loose on Monday tightened up on Tuesday. Now, *if* I pay attention, I find that not one thing in one day is identical to anything the day before or after it. If I don't pay attention, days and years run together, and I run the risk of posing that deadliest of questions, "Where did all the time go?"

Stories and poems are about changes. The majority of the time we have is made up of subtle changes, not catastrophic ones. It's the daily shifting of perspectives, allegiances, even clothing that make us who we are. Lives are a melding of small shifts, and your stories must contain these small shifts. A writer must be tuned in to the subtleties of change, or else his work will always be about catastrophes. Yes, sometimes there's death, hurricanes, a broken heart, but you can't stack your plot with a series of Red Alert disasters. You have to be attuned as well to subtlety. We notice this subtlety first in our own lives. Our own flesh. Pay attention. There are stories to hear in your bones, your flattened arch, your first age spot. The ease through which you breathe in one nostril compared to the other. The tightness or softness of your throat when you swallow. Every day, every minute, subtly shifting.

In our post-Industrial age, most of us have lived our lives

surrounded by very efficient machines. The machines perform, day after day, in exactly the same way, because that's what machines do. This consciousness has seeped into our expectations for ourselves when it comes to our work process. We expect that we can achieve the same level and depth of work every single day. We are not machines. We are organic matter, subject to any number of inconsistencies—physiological, emotional, psychological—that keep us from producing the exact number of words with the exact level of focus today as we did yesterday. We are human and imperfect and constantly changing, and we must allow for that change in our creative lives.

Follow the storms of your own changing weather patterns to see what is on the other side. Don't hold out for seventy-two degrees and sunny before you write. Write when it's raining, too, realizing that visibility might be less than on a sunny day, but that you might notice something amazing in the puddle you stepped in that you'd have never seen with your sunglasses on. Be flexible. Rather than resist the blizzard, see what you notice when you're in it. Pay attention. When the snow melts, pay attention. Live and observe each moment of your lives. Notice the ebbs and flows, the ultimate pattern of events.

As you fine-tune your observation skills to notice the subtle shifts in your own view of the world, branch out with those skills into the world of your fiction and poetry. The subtleties lend believability. They cultivate intimacy with the reader. They allow the reader to trust you, so that when he settles into his chair with your book in his hand, he'll say, "Yes. This writer is *present*." And that's all there is to it, really. Cultivate an awareness and appreciation of the present moment and notice how you can't help but move that into your writing. Where you are, your writing will be. Energy follows consciousness. Pay attention. In just a second, it'll all be different.

Touchstones

1. Keep a "body journal." Each day, notice the sensations in your body. Be very specific. Don't just say, "My back hurts." Find out (and get an anatomy book if you need to) which vertebrae are affected. Don't just focus on areas of pain or discomfort. We tend not to notice our bodies if they aren't causing us any trouble. Pay attention as well to the parts that are free from pain and are working perfectly.

2. Make a list of what is different today from yesterday. These can be more than just physical things. Do this practice for seven days. What do you notice?

3. What did your character *almost* do that would have changed everything? Write the scene of that moment of decision.

4. Freewrite on this prompt: To be wounded means . . .

20

SUFFERING

You know quite well, deep within you, that there is only a single magic, a single power, a single salvation . . . and that is called loving. Well, then, love your suffering. Do not resist it; do not flee from it. It is your aversion that hurts, nothing else.

HERMANN HESSE

WE SUFFER, PLAIN AND SIMPLE, when we want our experience to be something other than what it is. We suffer when we succumb to desire because we believe that attaining that desire will result in a permanent positive change. There's a faulty premise at work in that thinking. Everything is impermanent. Everything that has a beginning has an end. Everything that is born will die. The feeling we have today of joy will change to sorrow and will change again to joy. We are not stagnant beings. Yet, we suffer profoundly because of our belief that we can somehow freeze and hold moments we enjoy forever and not participate fully in moments that cause us discomfort. This is not a cycle we can win. The sooner we can accept transience as a given, the sooner we can access our deepest voices.

There are many ways suffering of this nature manifests itself in writing. The most obvious way is the belief that a particular outcome or achievement (winning that prize, getting that fellowship, finding an agent) will result in continued happiness and bliss. It won't. But as long as you think it will, you'll stay on the wheel. It is cool to win a prize or get published or find an agent, but those things are also impermanent.

Another place this type of suffering shows up is in the actual writing itself. You're going along great and suddenly you become obsessed with finding a particular fact about life in fourteenth-century Spain and the writing stops. You scour the Internet. You may even go to the library. You're focused. You're on a mission. But what you've really done is given all your energy to a distraction that ultimately, like an itch, will only offer momentary satisfaction once it's quelled. Notice the next time you feel an itch on your body. Don't scratch it. Notice how the more you don't scratch it the more it acts like it is ripping your leg apart. Don't scratch it. After awhile, when your mind realizes you're not going to accommodate that itch, it moves on to something else. The trauma that was the itch becomes a nonissue, which it was all along. I'm not telling you never to scratch, but I am asking you to notice where the metaphoric itches surface in your writing process. And I'm asking you, just one time, to not scratch. Notice what happens next.

A third way suffering manifests in writing is when the writer attempts to control the work. This is linked to that desire for a particular outcome. The key to recognizing this stumbling block is the phrase "I want my character to . . ." Wherever you hear yourself beginning something connected to your writing with "I want," pay attention. You're entering the never-ending ego zone. You've preset an agenda and you're going to be dissatisfied if you allow yourself to write deeply,

letting the characters speak to you, and find they go in a different direction than you planned. If you already know where
you're going, then the journey is forced, choppy, and predict-
ably direct. You don't have to know so much. You don't have
to be the boss of everything. Just like you don't have to hold
up the whole world. You can lay it down for awhile. The world
will keep turning. Witness your stories. Don't direct them.
After they've found their own direction and voice, you can
tighten them up, massage the plot, develop more tension. But
don't do that before you have the material to do it with. Attempting to control your writing is a surefire recipe for suffering.

A fourth way we experience suffering in our writing is the
false belief that writing originates from thinking. "Of course it
does!" you may be saying. "I must think about something before I can write about it!" But that's not entirely the case. Our
minds do, of course, participate in the writing process. If my
brain were not functioning, I would not be able to type these
words into my computer. I would not be able to breathe or sit
upright. All of us have thoughts. But we are *not* our thoughts.
Ten minutes sitting on a meditation cushion will show you
the "thought chaos" going on in your mind at any given time.
When we try to follow our thoughts, they vanish. When we
try to follow our thoughts without judgment or attachment,
they fall away into other thoughts and ideas. When we don't
hold on to thoughts we remain unaffected by them. But what
are our thoughts? What are we? Who is witnessing the
thoughts? How can we be in intimate communion with something we observe if we are not that which we are observing? I
don't know. It's a puzzle all of us are working out in our own
ways.

I encourage you to try a practice of not identifying with
your thoughts; instead, watch them with amused detachment.

Marvel at what a crazy thing this human condition is! Let your thoughts flow through you like breath. Don't hold on to them longer than their lifespan of a moment. As you practice a flow with your breath and a flow with your thoughts, you will find it easier to enter the flow stage in your writing process.

You may have heard writers talking about being in the "zone." This is another way of referring to the state of flow. Athletes experience it. Painters experience it. You can experience it gardening, walking, or praying. We enter that flow state when we are completely present with whatever activity we are doing. Many writers speak of reading their work after writing it in the "zone" and feeling like they are reading someone else's work. They have no conscious memory of writing it. They just allowed the words to move through them onto the page. That place of flow, of trust, created the only thing it can—life.

You also experience suffering when you are dissatisfied with the work you've done today. You wanted it to be x, but it turned out to be y. What if y is really a stronger option? Or, what if y is the only way you can get to x, but you don't know that yet because you've stopped writing because x didn't surface right away. Give the writing space. Be patient. Keep showing up. Remain unattached.

The Buddhists tell us life is suffering. It is, but not because life is inherently awful, but because we, as human animals, continue to operate from an illogical premise. We suffer because we're attached to permanence and outcome. Work with that for awhile. Mull it over while you're on the wheel. Follow your thoughts back to their origin and discover they are nothing. Examine how much energy you've placed into believing your thoughts. Work with that for awhile and, more importantly, write about it for awhile.

We are human beings, so we will not be blissfully happy all

day, every day. Our writing process will not produce gems every time we sit down to the keyboard. Our relationships and our jobs will not always be what we want them to be. Don't try to move away from these truths. Move *into* them. They are also impermanent. You might as well explore every experience you're having as fully as you can. The next moment will be different.

Touchstones

1. Freewrite on this prompt: "Suffering means . . ."

2. Make a word cluster from some of the ideas in your free-write from number 1. Some examples of words might be: stuck, masks, freeze, fear, move, thoughts, scar, belief. Pick one of the words from your word cluster and freewrite on it. From that freewrite, find a specific image to illustrate your writing. On a new piece of paper, begin again, using that specific image to get you going.

3. Spend one of your writing practice periods writing down your thoughts exactly as you're noticing them. You'll see that the thoughts come faster than you can write. That's OK. Catch what you can. Don't censor the thoughts and don't try to make a coherent narrative out of them. The purpose of this exercise is just to notice what's happening in your head. Make sure to sit through an entire twenty-minute freewrite period to do this. Put it away for a few days and then go back and reread what you've written. What do you notice? How many topics do you cover? How much is linear? How much is circular? How much is un-identifiable or unintelligible? Again, the purpose is obser-vation, not judgment.

4. Remember a time when your thoughts and your thoughts alone created a mood for you. This could be something like scripting a potential confrontation at work that you fear will happen or worrying about the outcome of a problem in a relationship. The idea is to notice how your thoughts can create entire storylines around events that haven't happened, and may never happen, and from those thought patterns, how your energy changes. When you've got an example in mind, quickly write down the circumstances. Try to recreate the moment before your thoughts took over the narrative and the moment after your thoughts let go. From this piece of freewriting, compose a poem or prose piece about the adventure of your mind.

21

PERSEVERANCE

all at once like a flash flood of love, grace, and need,
the Heart finds its release

GUS BRETT

I OFTEN TEACH A three-semester-long novel-writing course. This is not for the faint of heart, nor is it for people who have a "plan." In some ways, the class is doomed to "fail" because writing a novel in three semesters is a little silly. Yes, you put one word after the other. How long can it take to write 75,000 words? But, as any writer will tell you, it's not how long it takes to write the number of words; it's how long it takes to put them in the right order. Because writing is such a personal process, there are no blueprints you can download to show you, step by step, how to put your book together. There are books that try. What they can offer is a formula for writing that will enable you to write the requisite number of words. But they can't tell you how to write *your* book. Nobody can. Each book will bring up its own issues for you. Each book presents its own struggles, themes, and dark areas in your heart. Each book will give you its voice and structure if you do the work. In my experience, the more consistent the "showing up" part of my writing process is, the more consistent the "writing" part of the process is.

Just because you accept the invitation doesn't mean the road will be smooth. You may have sleepless nights wondering what to do about John and Jane's affair in your novel. You may receive rejection after rejection from magazines, agents, and publishers. You might look out your window at a beautiful spring day and wonder why you are still sitting in front of your computer involved in the lives of imaginary people. Perhaps you'll find yourself obsessed with a story for three weeks and then find yourself disinterested for two months. Or, maybe you will read a novel that is so brilliant and original that you become stifled, knowing you will never measure up to that writing. You could be lured by seductive books, teachers, conferences, and academic programs. You might believe, momentarily, that the newest version of Microsoft Word will make your novel come together instantly and that high-speed Internet will make the research go faster. Your very bones may tell you that you have chosen the wrong project and that you must abandon it for a newer, more enticing one. But again, like a personal relationship, if you want to maintain it, you continue to show up, even when you'd rather be having coffee with the new gentleman from accounting. You continue to show up when the words don't come because you know they will return. You continue to show up because you know that without this relationship you are only a shell of who you could be. And you know this from the times you have abandoned it and then returned on your knees with flowers and candy to try to rekindle the fire.

No one can give you a tailor-made plan for your project because no one knows the things lurking in your shadow self. Not even you. So, when you start to write, you mine those shadowy places, often unconsciously, and find yourself face to face with what you don't want to look at. You are surprised by this (especially if you had a plan) and often get frustrated.

We mislabel this period in the process as writer's block. But it isn't a block. Not really. It's the discomfort that arises when we're put in situations we'd prefer to avoid. It's easier (or seems so at the time) to move away from the discomfort and start something new. I've worked with many students who are perpetual "starters." They have great ideas, get very excited about their projects, and then when it comes time to do the work, they stop at the first roadblock and have a new great and perfect idea. This cycle will get you as far as the hamster gets on his exercise wheel. What it will teach you, however, is what your tendencies are.

As writers, it's very important that we're aware of our own methods of distraction and avoidance. The more we become aware of them, the more we can consciously avoid them and stay with the work. As I've mentioned previously, online shopping is a huge distraction for me. Here I am, typing away on a project, and the e-mail flag pops up. Oh! A coupon for just what I need! It's even more appealing if I didn't know I needed it in the first place. So, I dive into the Internet (still during my writing time) and emerge poorer and frustrated with my work. Awareness of this distraction gives me an opportunity to watch what I do and why I do it so I can learn. We've all got "distractions of choice." The practice is not never be distracted. The practice is to pay attention. Notice when you do them. Become aware. Be *with* the discomfort. What would happen if you didn't turn away from the work right then? What would happen if you stayed?

In class, I give my students a prompt, watch them write three or four sentences, and then stop writing. I try to suggest that they keep writing even when they think they have nothing to say. I use Natalie Goldberg's "keep the pen moving" mantra. When we stop writing, we tend to stop well within the place of safety. We stop when we still feel in control. We stop when we feel the edges of something real biting at the pen. As writers, we must develop the ability to push through the urge to stop (or shop, or talk on the phone, or garden) and stay with what is emerging. Very rarely do we hit a bull's-eye on what we have to say the first time out. Part of this process of perseverance has to do with releasing the ego from the work. You're learning to let go of the "I"—as in "I want my character to do *x*" and "I want to write about racial inequality in America." You move through those initial desires and wants. Remember the ladder from chapter 9? Those desires may have gotten you to the desk, but it's time for them to go.

Many students come to a creative writing class with a capital *I* Idea. They are certain, beyond any shadow of a doubt, that they know exactly what they want to say and what they want the reader to take away from what they've said. This is OK. It's a beginning place. We all have to begin. So, their first drafts are ideas. They are very head based, not body based. They are full of pontifications, morals, and judgments. This is OK. We build from here.

Ideas in and of themselves are abstract. Good writing is specific. Concrete. Readers need something sensory to hang their hats on. So we continue to move deeper into the work. Give me an image for those abstract ideas, I'll say. Show me what you're talking about. We look for concrete language. Instead of "Susie is looking forward to school," we write, "Susie smoothes the wrinkles out of her new pink dress with tiny fingers. First grade begins today. She imagines the loops of the alphabet circling a classroom, joined by the points and angles of the numbers and the symbols, the plus sign, which looks like a cross, the take-away sign which looks like it lost a part, the pop of a period, the snake of the question mark and the sheer excitement of an exclamation point stretching from floor to ceiling with joy."

Now we're making progress. We move deeper still and start to think about who Susie is. What does she want? Why is she in my story? What does she sound like? Continuing on: "She knows today makes her a big girl. It moves her from one who is confined to the house to one who moves about in the world. She will learn things, things she cannot begin to imagine, and she will bring them home, and when mommy is passed out in the brown chair, a bottle of liquid, the same brown color as the chair and of mommy's hair when she washes it, nested in her hand, she will share what she's learned with daddy and maybe together they will know enough to run away." Ah. We've now got a problem, a conflict, and a motivation. Susie has a desire. We may be getting close to the heart. The longer we linger here, the more we'll discover. Maybe we'll find out that Susie really isn't the protagonist of our story. Maybe we'll have to cut Susie out entirely. It's OK. She got us to where we need to be. If we don't linger, hang around, loiter, *persevere*, we'll never know.

It's human nature to want to move quickly to the heart of the writing, but it takes discipline and perseverance to reach it. There simply is no way *around* the work. No shortcut. No fast track. No super-value meal method to the finish line. You can make up any number of games to distract yourself from the work. Believe me, I've done my share, but the bottom line is the bottom line. The work must be done and you must do it. No one else can write what you have to write. No one else sees the world exactly the same way as you do. No one else has the exact same fire in her belly as you do. Go ahead. Try to find a shortcut. You have to try to do that anyway, before you'll believe me that there isn't one. Try to write that novel in thirty days, three hours a day. Works about as well as trying to lose thirty pounds in thirty days (without of course, doing the work of exercising and eating less). Let me say it again. *There is no way around the work.* Your job is to find *your way* of being with the work. It can't be my way, or your mom's way, or your spouse's way. It has to be your way. You're cutting your own path through this forest. It simply cannot be any other way and sustain you.

You will not wake up one day and say, "Ah ha! I have reached deep writing!" and then go back to sleep. You will not get a gold star of accomplishment from the Deep Writing Intensive Correspondence Course. You will gradually notice that your writing has made an organic shift. You may still be working with the same stories or facing the same problems when you go to do your writing for the day, but your perspective on the problems will have shifted. Because you have used writing as a practice, you know that what is coming up for you today is just what is coming up for you today. It is not a sign from the universe that you should stop writing forever, nor is it a sign that you will win the Nobel Prize. It just is what it is. Because you know that you will never be "done" with your writing life, you will never run out of things to learn about it, ways to experiment with it, or opportunities to grow from it, you are no longer hung up on grants, prizes, and publication. You are walking the writer's path, taking the detours, backward steps and leaps of faith required to maintain the relationship with your writing that is a constant in your life.

In my novel-writing series, the second semester is focused on producing pages. I call it the "Texas period." I grew up in the east, where states fit in the palm of your hand. When we moved west, it seemed to my young mind that all of New England could fit in New Mexico. Apparently it can, and nothing has yet to compare to crossing Texas (and we only crossed the panhandle). It seemed appropriate, as I began to work with larger and longer pieces of writing, to somehow come to terms with this "middle" space where the enthusiasm of beginning has waned, but the end is not in sight, and you really, truth be told, have very little idea of what you've got to work with (though you're sure it's junk). The way I came to terms with it was to think about that drive through Texas. It felt like a black hole. We crossed into it, but we never crossed out of it. We passed a graveyard of Cadillac cars upended outside of Amarillo that has haunted me. People don't make it out of here, I thought. People get stuck; they dehydrate and fossilize. There's little moisture, so they don't rot. They turn to paper and blow away. Ask anyone who's stuck through the process of writing a novel and they'll recognize the "Texas period." They may call it something else, but they've all been there and they've got the battle scars to prove it. Keep moving. Don't stop and become food for turkey vultures.

Everything that has a beginning has an end. You entered Texas and you will leave Texas if you keep the car fueled and maintained and keep yourself pointed west (or east), toward the ocean. Keep your body fueled and maintained. Eat, rest, play, dream. But write. Mile by mile, word by word, and in the famous words of Anne Lamott, "bird by bird," you'll get out and the beauty of the Rockies will leave you breathless.

Touchstones

1. What tricks have you tried to make the writing "easier"? What worked or didn't work with them?

2. Make a map of your "Texas period." Where are you now? What do you need to do to get through?

3. Can you identify the heart of your work? Articulate it with an image. Don't despair if you can't yet. You will.

4. Are you tired of your project? If so, give yourself a break for a week. Then, return to it with fresh eyes. Write about your experience of being separated from the work.

5. Explore the notion of "being lost." What does that bring up for you? How does it relate to your writing?

6. What passages have you been through? Where have you gone alone to find yourself? Write about them.

PART THREE

EMBRACING WHAT AND WHERE YOU ARE

Do not try to become anything.
Do not make yourself into anything.
Do not be a meditator.
Do not become enlightened.
When you sit, let it be.
What you walk, let it be.
Grasp at nothing.
Resist nothing.

AJAHN CHAH

You've just finished your novel. You release a sigh from your belly, deep, low, and long. You exhale, smile, save your file, look around your office, and then . . . what? Where did everybody go? And for that matter, *who* are you if you're not working on that novel you've been carrying with you in your body for decades? Completing a project you've been living with for years is often unsettling, strange, and empty. After the glow of accomplishment fades, you are left with only you, your breath, and space. It's highly likely that no one ever told you about this space, and if they did, they didn't tell you how to be with it.

Our final section helps you recognize *when* you're in this place between projects and *how* to embrace it and learn from it. All writers who see a project through to completion will find this place, though it looks different to each writer. Part 3 shows you how to find the gifts available to your writing and to you as a writer by remaining still, emptying your body fully of your project, and waiting. Writers must detach from their old work so that there is space for new work to enter. We can't fill ourselves with new stories until we have released completely the stories we've been working on. There just won't be room.

Many writers experience a period of letdown or grief after a project is completed. They may miss their characters. They may worry they'll never have another idea again. Being able to hold here, your last novel on the ledge behind you, next novel not yet visible in front of you, requires courage. It requires patience, balance, and compassion, surrender and stillness.

This "middle passage" is not a time of inactivity and laziness, though it may look that way on the surface. You're not writing anything. You're not sure what you want to be working on. You don't feel inspired. But rather than being a place of "nothing," it is the beginning of a bridge to your next idea.

Part 3 will guide you through the letting-go process. It will help you bid farewell to your project and clear out a place for the next one. It will help you breathe, unencumbered by what you have been writing and by what you will be writing.

Close your eyes now, and jump.

Body Break

This is a fun breathing activity for letting go. It's sometimes called lion breathing. Stand with your feet slightly more than shoulder width apart. Bend your knees slightly and place your hands on your thighs. Inhale and scrunch up your face as tightly as you can. Close your eyes and press your lips together. It's OK if it feels goofy. Clench your whole body as tightly as you can. Count to three and release with a roaring sound, opening your mouth wide and sticking your tongue out as far as you can.

Why? It releases facial tension, stimulates the free flow of lymph, opens the center of communication (throat chakra), and helps promotes smooth function of the thyroid and parathyroid. It also can make you laugh, which in and of itself is a great release!

22

IMPERMANENCE

The life which is dying is existing right here now and is grateful.

ZEN WISDOM

EVERYTHING THAT BEGINS, ENDS. There are no exceptions to this rule. This is the only guidance I can give you that I can't find an exception to. I remember when I was very young and first becoming aware that everything dies. I remember also being completely unable to comprehend myself not being alive. How sad, I thought, that everything dies in the world. *"Except me,"* I added softly. It went without saying that I would outlive everything. I don't know if others feel that way at certain points in their development. I still wrestle with that tiny voice that says *except me*. I still believe there's a very deep part of me that is certain I will escape death. But I won't. And you won't either.

Working with impermanence will deepen your writing practice. Let me break it down into two categories for you. The first is the impermanence of your own body and life. The second is the impermanence of your writing. "But wait!" I can hear you scream. "Writing is forever!" Just hang in there with me for a minute. I'll explain what I mean.

First, you must look at your own impermanence. As writers, you're constantly being pulled into the parts of your soul that others stay away from. You're digging deep in the recesses of your own shadowland. This is the first myth I want to debunk: No matter what your little voice says, your time is limited. You don't know how limited it is. It's dangerous to assume you'll live healthfully to a ripe old age. You just don't know. Armed with that knowledge, the moments that you are living right now are precious and fleeting.

I went back to school to get my MFA when I was thirty. In our first opening circle, a man in his late fifties was there. He was very excited to be in the program and to be devoting his time to his writing. He'd been waiting for this his whole life. He finally had enough money in the bank, time to take off from his job, kids established in their own lives. It was time for him. He didn't come to the next class. Or the next. Turns out, as you might have suspected, he died in his room of natural causes. Even though we did not know him, his death sent a deep shock wave through our group. The up-close-and-personal intellectual realization: *that could have been me.* Then, the real heart of that realization: *one day that will be me.*

The urgency that naturally accompanies a brush with death is normal. But we can't construct a writing life based on fear. The "ohmigod, I've got to finish this novel *today* because I might die tomorrow" will only result in raising your blood pressure. And the "I've got all the time in the world—I'll start tomorrow" will only result in your not starting at all. What's the balance? Acceptance of your own impermanence. I'm not going to pretend that if I found out tomorrow I was dying, I wouldn't bargain and do everything possible to stay here. But I also know that I am dying. Right now. And so are you. We just don't have a date. A meditation on impermanence will help you come to terms with that. I have a favorite mantra:

Everything that has a beginning has an ending.
Make your peace with that and all will be well.

Try meditating on that a few times a week. See what shifts occur for you. We can't write twenty-four hours a day. But we can begin to think about the time we have differently. Time is a concept created by humans. Time is undisturbed by our desires. We can neither bargain with it nor run from it. It moves at the same pace for all of us. The variable is our perception of the time. The variable is our relationship to the time and our awareness of it.

When I visited Rome, I went to the Capuchin crypt, which is located beneath the seventeenth-century Capuchin Church of the Immaculate Conception near Barbarini Square. The Capuchin monks made dioramas and sculptures from the bones of the monks within their order. They didn't kill the monks, but as a monk died, his bones became part of the sculptures. There are many theories as to why they did this, but the result is an astonishing underground assembling of bones into chandeliers, chairs, beds, clocks, and other skeletal figures. Some say the monks used this as a meditation on impermanence. Whatever the original reason, one can't view this crypt without contemplating mortality.

I found the crypt to be breathtakingly beautiful. Not in a gee-I'd-like-to-have-that-on-my-wall sort of beauty, but a deeper beauty. The monks, to me, created a space where we could witness the precious vulnerability of the human body. We could view, in the bones of others, what we will never be able to see in ourselves. We walk around in these bodies, but we don't know what they look like on the inside. We wouldn't be able to pick out *our* femur or *our* collarbone from a dozen others. The crypts show us that we are fragile, beautiful, and far more similar than we may like to imagine.

Now, on to the writing. Some people come from a background where it was never safe to write anything down. Your parents might read it. Or your older brother. Your very words could incriminate you. Some of us have learned to keep our words secret to protect ourselves or others. Words have power. I'm not going to try and argue that once you put something down on paper it stays there; there's not much point to that. But I would like you to consider the idea of impermanence as it relates to your work in the context of detachment.

Let's first define terms. When I speak of detachment, I don't mean you no longer care about the work, or that you didn't care when you were writing it. I don't mean detachment in the Western psychological sense of being unable to form healthy relationships or engage in the world. Detachment has a negative connotation in Western psychology. Likewise, attachment has multiple meanings depending on the context. In Western psychology, we talk about the importance of forming attachment bonds. In Buddhism, we talk about the perils of attachment. The concept of detachment that I am referring to deals with detaching from our unhealthy attachments. Detachment, at its heart, centers on an awareness of the impermanence of all things.

I know it can be challenging to think about detaching from something you have created. It may seem even stranger if you haven't yet completed a project. But if you want your work to be read by others, whether a friend, a critique group, or a publisher, you'll find the experience far less painful if you've learned to cultivate a healthy detachment. Here are three ideas to help you work with this concept.

1. You are not your work. As Americans, we identify heavily with our employment. When we meet people, we often ask, "What do you do?" And they answer, "I am a doctor, a teacher, a dancer." Those statements are only partially true.

Let's look deeper into those phrases and see what's at the heart of them. A doctor heals. A teacher teaches. A dancer dances. But is a doctor the medicine he prescribes? Is a doctor the diagnosis she delivers or the surgery she performs? Is a teacher his lesson plans? Her final exam? Is a dancer the individual choreographed steps? As a writer, are you the words on the page?

Yes, you are a writer. A writer writes. You write, every day perhaps. You write when you'd rather be doing just about anything else. Still you show up. Yes, you are a writer. But you are not your novel or your poem any more than a doctor is her prescription for penicillin. The sooner you can learn to release your work, the sooner you will be able to integrate yourself with the flow of the work. When you hold on to it, you create blocks for yourself. You worry about the outcome. You try to force a resolution. You may worry about how you will be perceived by writing the story. Don't give energy to those thoughts. There is plenty inside you. You won't run out of stories to write. This is what you do, right? You write. So, write. Release. Write. Release. Just like breathing.

2. You cannot control the outcome of your work. When I use the word outcome here, I'm not talking about whether or not you can make a novel or a poem, though sometimes you'll find the stories definitely dictate their own terms to you. I'm talking about publication, reviews, product placement, advertising, remaindering, talk show bookings, textbook adoptions, and any and all manner of what happens to the work after you write it. You can help yourself by being actively involved in self-promotion of your work. You can help yourself by making phone calls, giving readings, and educating yourself as much as possible about the business of publishing. Don't sit idly by after you sign your contract and let the publisher handle everything. Be aware of the ins and outs of the business. Ask

intelligent questions. Be engaged in your own success. But understand that you can do all those things and still find your book on the remainder table. Lots of books are printed every year and lots of books are remaindered every year. Lots of books are sold and lots of books get bad reviews. You can't change this. What you can do (say it with me again) is write. Keep writing. Keep yourself focused on what you're currently working on. Maintain a healthy involvement in the business end of your work, but don't worry about the business end until you have a product to sell. Once you have a product to sell, do your homework. And remember that whatever will be, will be. If you hang your feelings of success on a good review, you'll have to hang your feelings of failure on a bad one. Both are out of your control. Both will happen regardless of what you do. Write the book. Let it go. Write the next one.

3. You cannot control people's perception of your work. This is really the heart of the detachment process. Think back to any literature class you've taken. If there were twenty students in the class, there were probably twenty different perceptions of *The Grapes of Wrath,* none of which was likely Steinbeck's interpretation. In Amy Tan's memoir, *The Opposite of Fate: Memories of a Writing Life,* she talks about reading the Cliff's Notes to *The Joy Luck Club* and wondering what book the authors had read.

It's not our job to interpret our work for the world. That doesn't mean that it isn't our job to make that work as clear, concise, precise, and engaging as possible. There's no excuse for vague writing. But the writer is engaged in a triad of writer, writing, and reader. As writers, we are but one piece—one leg. The writing, the work, is another piece, and the reader completes the trinity. Once the reader is involved, the magic of the paradox of permanence and impermanence reveals itself. Yes, the words remain the same on the page, but the ideas and feelings the reader takes from those words are as varied as fish in the sea. As writers, we not only have to be OK with that, we need to embrace that as part of the organic nature of art. You will not be able to control how other people respond to your work. You will not be able to control what they choose to interpret about it, what they choose to label it, or how they choose to receive it. Accept these things early in your writing career and it will go easier for you.

Think about your own experience with a book. Have you ever read something, say in high school, and thought it was the most brilliant book in the world, then reread it when you were in your thirties and wondered what you could have possibly seen in the book? None of the words in the book have changed. They are the same as when you first read it in ninth grade. The variable is you, the reader. That's as it should be. Pick the book up again in your eighties and see what you think. The text remains, but the response to the text changes. You cannot control this. Focus instead on what you can do, now, today, and all that is (and it is enough) is to write. So, get busy. The rest is not up to you.

Touchstones

1. Write a poem about the things/people/beliefs that are no longer a part of your life.

2. Your protagonist is seconds from death. What is the one thing she wishes she had said or done? What would be different about the plot of your story if this had occurred? How does the "not doing" of this thing affect the plot?

3. Write two monologues. Begin one with, "Yesterday I lost . . ." Begin the next one with, "Today I found . . ."

23

EVOLUTION

Notice that the stiffest tree is most easily cracked, while the bamboo or willow survives by bending with the wind.

BRUCE LEE

WHAT DO YOU MEAN I've got to do it all over again? I spent five years on that novel draft! I am so sick of it I can't stand it. I've got this better, fascinating, more captivating idea for the next book though, and I just want to get moving in that direction—away, away, away, from this project. Sound familiar?

In my teaching experience, nothing evokes the blank, "fish eyes" response from a class faster than talking about revision. They lift their heads from text messaging long enough to wonder what they've gotten themselves into. A single paper wasn't enough? They have to do it again? And not just fix the punctuation? I'll admit, when I was in college algebra, I didn't want to do anything over. I wanted the answer, but if I didn't get the answer, that was OK because I was never going to use higher math. So, I know many of my students are often in this same place. But, people who claim they *want* to be writing and want to be writers should not balk at the idea of revision. What is the value of revising something? Why isn't the first time "good enough"? And what do we really mean when we talk about revising a story or poem?

Let's first talk about what we're *not* talking about. You're not just going through and deleting (or adding) the commas. That's final editing, and yes, it is part of the larger revision stage, but it's not the behemoth "oh my god I've got to do it again" revision that every project must go through. Get the high school English teacher red pen out of your mind and think about imagination. That's right. Imagination. (See, there's some moon energy, some right-brained energy in this part, too!)

It might be helpful for you to break the word apart. Re-visioning. You are looking at your work anew, with fresh eyes, innocent eyes, from a place of humility and curiosity. Your first draft has given you a piece of the work—a door into deeper possibilities. Now you get to focus. You get to find the heart of your characters and your work. You've got a spring-board now (and nothing that you wrote in the first draft is wasted—absolutely nothing), and you can stretch yourself, moving deeper into the work while still remaining grounded in the skeleton of the story.

The revision stage is a wonderful place to work with the conflicting energies inside you. You get to experience the stretching—the reaching forward and out, while at the same time reaching back and down, rooting your feet in the process and development of the piece.

Notice I didn't say you've rooted your feet in the first draft. You've got to move through that first draft. If you stay anchored to it, it'll sink you. Here's a place where writers get stuck. They feel they have to stay attached to what they just wrote! After all, it took so much to get *that*—what will they do without it? This is normal thinking, but it doesn't serve you or your work. Remember I said there are no shortcuts to this writing thing? I really did mean it. You have to write the early drafts to find the heart of the work. Early drafts lead to final drafts. You don't start with a final draft. It's arrogance, laziness, or complacency that gets writers thinking that they don't need to follow this process all the way through. Writers revise. Period.

Body Break

Stand in mountain pose (see chapter 2). Pay attention to your feet. Feel all four corners of your feet pressing into the earth. Slowly raise your arms above your head, fingertips pointing toward the sky. As you reach your arms toward the sky, continue to be aware of your feet pressing down toward the earth.

Why? This pose gives you the opportunity to observe this reaching and rootedness within your own body.

The more organically you can imagine the process of creating a piece of writing, the easier it will be for you to release rigid definitions of prewriting and revision. There's an ebb and flow on both sides, and yes, sometimes one crosses the line into the other. Be as open to these fluctuations as you are to the sudden departures and arrivals of your characters. The well fills up when the water is released. If nothing is released, nothing enters.

Revision is a chance for you to rethink, reimagine, and most importantly redream your work. You've gotten some pieces out. Maybe some will fit the final puzzle. Maybe none will. But *all of them* worked to get you to this place. Honor them. They are not wasted words or wasted efforts. You might think of this revision place as the Olympic ski run. You've done the bunny hill stuff. Now, you're ready to see what you've really got. It's OK, too, if you find you don't have much of anything. That's also part of the process. Sometimes you have enough meat to make a sandwich; sometimes you've got to go shopping. It's OK. A piece of a discarded draft can haunt you for years, eventually turning into your first novel once you've experienced what you needed to experience to write that story. Sometimes our characters are farther ahead of us than we're comfortable with and it takes some time to catch up. That's why this is a process that we have to surrender to and trust. We don't know everything, and thank goodness, because if we did, we'd have way too many ideas and characters to explore and write about.

After you feel like you've got a pretty decent early version, you might seek out feedback from a teacher or writing group. You want to avoid feedback too early in the process because then your ideas get wrapped up with other people's ideas before the work has a chance to get its sea legs. The birth of a story is a fragile time and should be treated as such. But sooner or later, your baby will have to go out in the world and the world will have its way with it. Get used to that.

After you receive feedback from competent readers, read everything over again and make your own decisions about what feedback is going to work for you and what isn't. Don't try to incorporate everything a dozen people said for you to do. You'll wind up with nonsense. Competent readers can be found in colleges, bookstores, and local writer's groups. Generally, unless your spouse or parent has the education or publication record to support their opinions, they're not much help because they love you. You need readers with an objective eye, ones who are literate in the craft of creative writing and capable of clearly articulating what they mean to say and, more importantly, *why* they are saying it. A good reader is worth his or her weight in gold.

You have to learn to be a good reader, too, so you can help other writers and learn to read your own work more objectively. Being a good reader doesn't mean you read ten books a month. Being a good reader means you are able to understand the craft choices an author made and ascertain whether or not they worked and why. A good reader is familiar with the terminology, the lingo, of the field. He knows the forms of dialogue. He knows what narrative tension is and how to put it there when it's missing. He understands the difference between a character arc and a narrative arc. He had to learn these things, and you do, too, because you want to be a good writer, and in order to do that, you must learn your craft. Many of the books listed in the appendix can help you with this, but you really learn your craft by practicing your own writing and by reading the works of others. You can't be an architect without learning all the tools of the building trade. You can't be a musician just because you bought a guitar and strummed it a few times.

Knowledge is power, and in no other place is it more apparent that knowledge is missing than in the revision stage. I think many writers freak out here because they don't know exactly *how* to do anything more than they've done. They may not even be sure of what they've done yet. This is normal, too. Everyone begins at his or her own beginning. You come to writing because you have a drive to do it. Then you find there's more to learn than you ever thought possible, but you want to be here in this field with these people, so you learn. Then you find you're never done with the learning, but you stay anyway. Your early drafts merge into final, publishable drafts. Your initial ramblings and confusions take on direction and confidence. You've stayed with the work, and the perseverance will be rewarded.

So, yeah, yeah, but what do I *do* now? The first thing to do is reread your first draft and then put it away. Yes, put it away. Breathe it in, hold it for a minute, and then let it go. Let all of it go. Put it in a drawer. Hide it in a computer file. But get it out of your eyeball range. I can hear the gulps from here. Trust me on this. Holding on to it is going to stifle the next phase. You've got what you've written inside of you. You know what you've done. You know who your characters are. You know what scenes you particularly liked or didn't like. You know what part of this early draft is continuing to call to you and pull you in. You know these things because you're a writer. Now is the time to trust yourself. Just pretend to trust yourself if you can't yet bring yourself to buy into what I'm asking you to do. Put it away and start again, re-seeing, re-visioning, redreaming. Start where the energy pull is. Start where there's still that nagging question about a character. Start where there's a problem with the image or metaphor or with a completely different character as the protagonist. Just start again and write until it's done. Then, do it again. And again. And again. And one of these drafts is going to shout at you, "Hey! I'm it! I'm it!" You'll know it. And when you hear that with your inner voice, that's the draft you edit. That's the draft on which you fix the punctuation, rebreak the paragraphs, and align the plot components.

It's OK if you don't believe me. Try it with a few stories or poems. I've seen it work time and time again with my students, most of whom fought me to the bitter end. I've seen it work with my own writing. It works because we have been so trained to focus on the "fixing" of things (as if your writing is broken) that when we see a very imperfect early draft, our mind zeroes in on the flaws because it's been trained to find them. Oh, there! Comma splice! Oh, there—you spelled it Chuckie in the first paragraph and Chucky in the seventh paragraph. Oh, no transitions! Oh! Oh! Oh! And before you know it, you've got a mess of metaphoric red ink on a piece of work not meant for the grammar police. It's like taking your brand-new baby, plopping him down in a doctoral program in quantum physics, and criticizing him because not only can he not understand the discussion, he can't even hold a pencil yet.

The mind will see what is in front of it and die trying to fix it. It will work with the components it has. The words you used the first time. The sentence structures. It will marry itself to what is in front of it, and subsequently shut off the creative flow, which is still necessary for the next steps. Your left brain will get terribly excited and want to get out the hacksaw. Not yet, not yet. You still need to be receptive, soft, and open. You still need to be able to listen to something other than your own thoughts.

Let's bring it into the body. Imagine you're trying to do a shoulder stand against a wall. You've positioned your blankets (i.e., your tools: notebook, laptop, pen) and you know what the end result is supposed to be because you see the teacher in the front of the class carrying on upside down like it's nothing. You grit your teeth (not recommended) and follow the step-by-step instructions he gives you for moving up the wall (first draft, beginner's mind, bird-by-bird). You see everyone around you going up like they were born that way (comparison to other writing students, published books) and you fall down.

You hope the teacher is aligning the other students who managed to get up and considers you a lost cause so you can be in peace until the next posture (let the best students get workshopped, praised, held up in the class so you can reinforce your ideas about yourself, and above all else, get yourself out of this uncomfortable place as soon as possible). But you're lucky (a word choice you might not use at the time). You've got a good teacher who comes over to you and says he can help you get up the wall. You've got a big choice here. You can say no because gosh darn it you don't want to be up the wall after all (who needs an agent and a book deal anyway), or you can recognize that right now, you can't get up the wall by yourself and he really could help you, and if he kept helping you, your body might one day find its way there all on its own. He sees what you can't yet see—that's what teachers do. And, if you kept trying to push into shoulder stand on the faulty foundation (early draft) you'd never get up because you weren't rooted in the real stuff yet. When your foundation is real, you bloom.

Just because you can pick up a pen or type doesn't mean you can write a perfect novel the first time out. You are always a student of your art and craft. You are always in a position to learn from others. The writer who is open to that, the writer who is honest with herself about her current limitations without judging them, the writer who is willing to fall on the floor in a room full of people, is the writer who will be left standing at the end of the day.

One of my favorite parts of any creative writing class comes at the end of the semester when I ask students to write me an essay about the revision process. I get to read about their struggles with what I've asked them to do and the joys they discovered even as they cursed me under their breath (or openly). I hear the childlike glee when one of their characters "took over" and their story opened up into someplace they never saw coming. It's a gift to participate in this process with them, and once you've done it yourself a few times, you'll find that you can survive it. Maybe you'll find you even thrive in it.

Writers revise. You're a writer. Open your eyes and see anew. Be willing to amaze yourself. Be willing to stretch in both directions at once. You won't pull apart; you'll break open into a rainforest of unexpected, gorgeous, messy life.

Touchstones

1. Write a process essay about a piece you've recently revised. What steps did you go through? What resistances did you face? What joys did you experience? How different was the finished piece from the earlier draft?

2. Examine a piece you're currently working on. Rewrite it using a different point of view. Change the setting and see what happens. Even changing the verb tenses from past to present or present to past affects the story deeply. Play with re-visioning. Let it be a dance.

3. Make a list of elements in your story that still excite you. Then make a list of elements in your story that no longer excite you. Don't make any changes yet, just observe.

4. Examine how either your writing process or your particular project has evolved since you began. What were your early beliefs about it? What is different now? What is the same?

24

SURRENDER

The end of all our exploring will be to arrive where we
started
And know the place for the first time.

T. S. ELIOT

I HAVE A VERY WELL-DEVELOPED EGO, both in the
Freudian sense and the vanity sense. I have healthy boundaries. I know I am not my mother, my partner, my job. But I
also know the ego's trappings. The way it manifests situations
to serve its needs. The way it hankers to keep the status quo.
The way it fights, for its very life, the notion of surrender. Yet,
if we are moving into authentic writing, we find ourselves face
to face with the imperative of "surrender."

Warning: Don't think for a moment this will go down
smoothly.

Let's examine the framework first and define some terms.
I'm not talking about surrendering to a "higher power" or
abdicating your personal power to any other being. I'm talking
about nothing less than surrendering your sense of self. Giving
yourself over to "anatta," which means "no-self" or "non-
self." I'm talking about dismantling the ego, the false self. It

will fight you every step of the way, and, I'll not mince words, it's easier to let it win.

But you've come this far, and this notion of surrender is so important to your development as an authentic writer, and for that matter, an authentic human, that I'll ask you to at least keep reading this chapter, even if you're doing what I have done—digging your heels in and screaming, "No! I will never surrender!"

Why do we need to surrender as part of the writing process? And doesn't "surrender" by definition, mean we have to surrender *to* something? Don't we have to subjugate ourselves to something else? No. What you need to do is strip away, piece by piece, the trappings of your false self. There's no quick trip through this. We have many stories in our global mythologies about this "stripping away" process. In Sumerian mythology, as Inanna descends to the underworld, she sheds something of value at each step along the way until she arrives, naked in the purest sense, ready to be reborn. Christ is stripped of his ego through physical suffering. The Buddha through unrelenting encounters with himself under the bodhi tree until he found "no self." We play with these stories, but most of the time we hang on the redemption end of them. We don't really want to dismantle our egos because we believe far too much is at stake.

In deep writing, which to me is a direct path to ego dismantling, we are faced with fairly predictable challenges as we set out on the writer's life. First, as beginning writers, we come to the page in a fairly settled egocentric space. By that, I mean that you think there is a "you" who is doing the writing, and that you (since you are in charge) can control your writing, and really *should* control your writing, thank you very much. You think writing is a task to complete. A checklist. But deep writing is a communication with unseen and intangible forces. It is an attempt to communicate, through stories, characters, and images that humans can understand, these unseen things. These unseen things are not hidden in the far reaches of planet Earth, but deep inside of your body. The deeper you go inward, the deeper your work becomes. You simply can't help it. As you journey inward, you find things you had no idea were there. How is that possible if you are in charge of you? Wouldn't you have at least some clue of what you've stored in your basement? As you discover more of yourself, you learn to release more of yourself, and then, in that space of emptiness, you write.

I often find quotes, books, films that speak to me though I don't know why at the time. I have stacks of books I haven't read, but the book I *need* to read is always here nearby. A few years ago I stumbled upon this gem. Unfortunately, I cannot find a source for it.

> To write what we are given to write,
> we must disappear.

I loved this quotation. I didn't understand it, but I loved it. I printed it out and put it on my wall above my computer. I had no idea *what* it meant, but I knew it said something important. I posted this quotation on one of my web-based creative writing classes. I used it as a journal prompt in different sections. I was enthralled by the responses I was getting, and I took note of the deep resistance my students displayed toward the concept. I've found that where there is resistance, especially a group resistance, to an exercise or an idea, there's some good stuff hiding!

After a few years of looking at the quote every day, I thought I figured it out. I thought it meant we had to get out of our own way (which we do). But that word *disappear* was a trigger word for me. Who wants to disappear? And if we disappear, who is doing the writing? And then, who am I? Am I even here at all? Aack! You can see the loop of questioning that this single quote can bring up. Here's the cold hard truth. People who live surface lives, people who swim in illusion, will write books and poems at that level. They will write things that communicate with other people who are at that level. Hopefully, they will come in contact with a teacher who whispers, "That's not quite it. Go deeper." The experienced teacher can spot a surface story. They're safe stories. Predictable stories. Stories without risk, either for the author or for the reader. The novice writer is often unaware that she has written a surface story. That's OK. The more she practices, the more she'll see—"Oh, yes, I pulled back here. Oh, I need to go deeper there. That's not yet the heart of the story." It's the *writing* that teaches us this. And it is the writing that pulls us in ever deeper. As you learn to trust the writing, you'll learn to release your attachment to the outcome. You'll learn to "disappear," literally, into emptiness.

Let's go back to the ego. The ego, also called the false self, is very strong. It is in business to survive and it is in business to keep you functioning in delusion. It wants you to write safe, sweet stories. It wants you to stay in previously explored territory. It wants to keep you on the straight and narrow. But the writing wants something else. The writing wants to release you. The writing wants to strip you, like Inanna, to your essence. And then it wants to erase you.

I know how terrifying that sounds. I know even how ridiculous it might sound. After all, I haven't addressed the earlier question of, if you go away, then who will be doing the writing? I'm not talking about killing your physical body. That's the farthest thing from this process. Your physical body is a gift to you. It houses all this amazing, uncharted territory. It is the vehicle through which you can express these things which can, ultimately, help shine some light on someone else's path.

To write what we are given to write, we must disappear.

In the physical practice of yoga, we take the time to sink deeply into positions of discomfort. We stay long enough to watch the distractions arise, get louder, get more persistent. Still, we stay. And one by one we release the distractions, and the pose, which once seemed impossible, is effortless.

If you allowed yourself to be stripped of your trappings, what would be left? This is surrender at its purest form. Not surrender to a higher power. Not surrender to another's belief system. Not surrender of your personal power. It is a surrendering of your self. There's no one else in the equation. Just you. And not you. Blow, and like a puff of smoke, you are gone. But you are not dead. You are awake. You are breathing. You are detached in a healthy way. You have disappeared. Now, what does that world look like to you? What stories, ideas, poems come from this boundless space? If you, as you have conceived of yourself, are not there, neither are the limitations and fears held by that "you." Your writing, unencumbered by ego's attempts to make it "be" something it isn't, make it "do" something it can't do, make it "say" something it can't say, is light and free and deep. Remember those times when you've reread what you've written the day before and asked yourself, "Where did that come from? I don't remember writing that."

Smile, then, and tip your hat. You disappeared into emptiness and brought back diamonds.

Touchstones

1. Take time to journal on the quotation, "To write what we are given to write, we must disappear." See what strikes

you. Let yourself go deeper and deeper into the words. What in the quotation scares you? What is intriguing? What raises questions? What are you most deeply resistant to?

2. Write a monologue beginning with: What is most stuck inside me is . . .

3. What patterns of suffering have you become accustomed to in your life? What would happen if you let them go? How do these patterns serve you? How do they cause you discomfort?

4. Think of an object in your life that you no longer need. The object should have emotional value for you. Write the story of how you came to have this object. Then take out that object. Look at it as if you've never seen it before. Notice its size, shape, color, and texture. Look at how it's made, what it did, what it does, and what it meant to you. Breathe naturally. Touch this object mindfully, with gratitude, honor and grace. Touch it with your eyes, touch it with your cheek, touch it intuitively with your eyes completely closed as well as with your fingers. Let yourself feel whatever it means to you. When you feel ready, let that object go. You can either give it away or bury it. After you've let it go, write anything that comes to you.

25

INTEGRATION

Unstiffen your supple body. Unchatter your quiet mind.
Unfreeze your fiery heart.

CELESTE WEST

PERHAPS BY NOW YOU'RE BEGINNING to see how many
hidden spaces and places there are within any task you choose
to perform. The surface level of things, with which we are
most inclined to identify, is just, as they say, the tip of the
iceberg. Say you take a class in writing dialogue that pops off
the page. You practice and you get pretty good. Then you take
a class on grammar and a class on characterization and a class
on internal rhyme. You'll end up with a lot of pieces—valuable
pieces for sure, but pieces nonetheless. We often focus on
gathering skills when we begin a new endeavor. I'll learn how
to stand properly. I'll learn how to point my feet. I'll learn
how to breathe. But then what?

Think back to when you were learning how to drive. Can
you remember how many things you thought you had to keep
track of? Turn the key, look behind you, keep your foot on
the brake, put the car in reverse, don't forget to keep looking
behind you (oh yes, and look in front of you at the same

time—it takes awhile to get the hang of the mirrors!). Now, you don't have to break down the skill of driving a car into its individual pieces. You get in the car, turn the key, and go. You've integrated driving into a flow.

This happens with writing too. When you first begin studying your craft, you may be very overwhelmed (are there really forty variations of third-person point of view?) with all the possibilities available to you. You may feel like you can never master them all, so it might be best to go back to watching TV. The first wonderful piece of news I have for you is that not only do you not have to master all of them, you won't, so no worries.

As artists, we are always growing and learning. We'll never reach the pinnacle of all we can learn about our art. Each piece we learn comes with its own puzzles and questions. Maybe you never knew there was such a thing as modulated dialogue. Maybe you always wrote dialogue based on sound. That's great, but if you know more about the finer points of dialogue, you can make more intelligent choices when you revise your piece. The more tools you have, the more integrated your structure will be. In this way, when you are in the prewriting stages, you're not pulling out your old class notes and thinking about the perils of adverb usage or the benefits of shorter paragraph structures. Instead, you'll be stepping outside yourself to that place of witness consciousness, the nonjudgmental space from which you pour out your stories. Then, in the revision stages, you go to your class notes, your textbooks, your toolbox, as Stephen King refers to it, and you consciously select what you need to suit the purpose of the work.

Two distinct parts of your brain are involved in this process. Your right brain gets to flow and leap and get crazy. Then, your left brain comes in and restores order so that others can share in the flow with you. These two forces that often push against each other need to find a way to live together, and in fact need to find a way to *nurture* each other, even as they continue to perform their separate functions.

If our goal is union, and if both of these parts are part of ourselves, then how can we bring them into greater harmony with each other? How do we integrate left and right, masculine and feminine, sun and moon? First, we honor the qualities of both. We recognize how each side contributes to a beautiful whole, and we see that without one of them, we would be unbalanced. How beautiful is the sky during the dawn and dusk periods where we can see both a sliver of sun and a shadow of moon? It's an almost otherworldly landscape that holds both equally—sun moving down into the west, moon rising in the east. Left-brained sun, right-brained moon.

Next, identify and accept your strengths and weaknesses. Don't say, "Oh, I know I really should be able to be more detail oriented (left brain)." It doesn't matter that you aren't naturally this way. Accept the truth of yourself. Then begin to experiment with characteristics and activities of the "other," (the side you're not overly comfortable with) always keeping in mind that there really is no other; you are always whole.

However, deeper integration is more than finding harmony between prewriting and revising. Deeper integration is a powerful surrender to the process you have participated in. It is the time when you exhale what you have gathered and release the product. You experience an unconscious coming together of the benefits of your work—your inspiration and your respiration. For example, each time you move into a yoga pose, your body reaps benefits. These are not always recognized that minute, that day, or that year, but subtle shifts are always occurring. Each time you finish a project, there is a time of integration where you recharge and ready yourself for the next venture, or inhalation. Because this often feels like doing "nothing," we have a tendency to move right through it. But it is a critical piece of the writing process because it provides the *time* and the *space* for the things you don't yet recognize to flourish.

I'd like to talk about integration in the context of the period that follows the "doing" of the writing itself. You've been on a roll. You've pumped out more pages than you thought possible. They're not even too bad for a beginning draft. You've surprised yourself with phrases and characters. You've learned much through the "doing." Here's where you want to stop. I don't mean pause to catch your breath. I mean a full stop. Before you jump to the next thing on your "doing" list, before you move into the next chapter, simply stop. Let the energy you've built up during this phase of writing spread throughout your body. Pay complete attention to this rush of energy moving through you. Stay present with it, and then allow yourself to focus on your third eye, that space between and just above your eyes. This is a place of unity and integration. You haven't finished. You're not resting yet. You're not in stillness. Focusing on your third eye will help merge the duality of energies within you. It will help you harmonize your process. Stay focused, aware, and awake. Breathe. This is as important as the "doing" you've just finished. Let all that you've done settle and find its natural place within you. You honor the good, solid work you've just done by letting it go. It's yours now. You won't lose it. Perhaps you're now beginning to know you've always had it.

Touchstones

1. What do you see are the qualities of the sun? The moon? How/where might these characteristics overlap each other? How do they serve one another?

2. What are some concrete ways you can integrate writing into your life? Don't think in terms of fitting in that six-week vacation. Think about a day-to-day incorporation.

3. Robert Pinsky said, "Poetry is a bodily art: its medium is not words or lives or images, or thoughts or ideas or 'creativity,' but breath, shaped into meaning in the throat and mouth." Freewrite on this quotation for fifteen minutes.

26

SOLITUDE

Loneliness is the poverty of self; solitude is the richness of self.

MAY SARTON

THE HUMAN BEING IS A SOCIAL ANIMAL. We like to be in communities. We like to form relationships. We thrive on physical contact from other human beings. By this point in the book, you've had ample opportunities to witness and experience the paradoxes of the writing process. It is a pull of opposites—a dance of desire and surrender. In previous chapters, I talked about the need for relationships—with your writing and with the world around you. This chapter addresses solitude, another part of the paradox. You can't "opt out" of the solitude part and expect to do much writing. You can't write a novel by committee. Even books written by two people aren't written by four hands on the same keyboard at the same time.

Don't, however, restrict yourself to a rigid definition of solitude. Just because you're a single mom with three kids doesn't mean you have to throw up your hands and cry you're never alone. Also, solitude doesn't necessarily mean you are by yourself. It doesn't require you to climb a fog-encapsulated mountain six hundred miles away from any other human. You don't have to have a second cabin in the woods. But you do have to create the space for solitude, and it will serve you better if you learn to cultivate it within your existing lifestyle, rather than hoping for that glorious moment when all distractions are gone, enough money is in the bank, and you no longer have that cramp in your leg.

Using a nonjudgmental eye, realistically examine your lifestyle. Are there fifteen minutes where you can go sit on the patio? Even going and sitting in the closet will work. This will give you a space where you can hear your mind. It'll be chaotic, likely a bit loud (and maybe dusty!), but that's OK. You're making space. If you live alone or without children, it may be easier to find the space, but there's a different set of challenges that surfaces. The grass isn't greener at either end of the spectrum. It's still grass.

Perhaps you've experienced what can happen when you finally secure that weekend alone to write. Maybe it's suddenly way too quiet. Or, way too loud. Maybe you find yourself unsure of what to do at first, so you make phone calls, go for a walk, or turn on the TV. Maybe it's the first weekend you haven't had the kids around in ten years, and on Saturday all you do is sleep. Then, the nagging voice begins. When are you going to write? See, you've given yourself this precious time alone and you still aren't doing anything. You'll never be a writer. And so, your grand plans collapse and you feel worse than you did before.

This scenario is not uncommon. We have to develop a relationship with solitude, just like we develop a relationship with people and with our writing. Otherwise, solitude itches. It feels like someone else's skin. It's too tight. Small, frequent encounters with solitude will let you slip into that weekend alone just like your favorite robe. But if you don't know each other, it will take awhile for the skin to fit. It's worth the investment. You won't feel as uncomfortable in your writing time if you wear solitude like a cape. You can experience solitude in a café surrounded by people. You can access it in the subway and at your kitchen table. Practice the techniques of sensory withdrawal I gave you in chapter 15. One by one, shut off the distractions. And, by the way, distractions are everywhere. Sometimes the most powerful ones surface when you are in the places most quiet. You can always find a distraction, and the real ones aren't outside of you in the barking dog or honking horn. They're inside in the form of thoughts.

Another somewhat different kind of solitude I've experienced occurs when we come to the end of a project—a book of poems, a novel, an essay collection. You've spent quite possibly years with these characters and these themes. Your characters become a part of your life and you know them more intimately than most if not everyone else in your life. And then, when the final piece of the story arc is over, they leave.

When I finished *Lay My Sorrows Down*, I was not prepared for that leaving. I thought for some reason that the characters would leave when I was ready for them to leave. In retrospect, I have no idea why I thought that. They didn't come when I called, so why would I have any say over when they go? I have two pieces of advice here.

First, don't try to hold on to them. Exhale them fully, like your breath. They have to go because you can't revise and work on the structure with a character whispering in your ear, and because you need to make space for the next book or project. Students are often worried that if they finish their novel they won't have anything else to write, so they drag out the finishing, thus ensuring nothing new can move in. Let go so you can fill back up. Watch your reactions as you near the end of a project.

Second, mark the ending somehow with ritual. For me, a candle, some nag champa incense, a glass of wine, and some quiet time is a good way to mark the passing, but you can develop your own rituals that have meaning for you and your particular project. Include gratitude for the experience and the relationship. Put your pen down. Exhale. Pause. Inhale. Feel the fullness of your body, buoyed by breath.

The fiction-writing process, while unique for every writer, does at some level involve an elaborate world of make-believe. If we stick with the stories, we become skilled at entering and exiting that world as needed to complete our work. Some writers believe they create the world and the characters who inhabit that world, and some writers believe that they are the means through which the characters speak their truths. These writers respond to dreams, synchronicities, and intuition along the writing path.

I don't know who is right, but I know which type of writer I am. As soon as I sit down and think I know where I'm going with a story, the characters stop talking to me. They go back to wherever they come from and I am left alone to direct a cast of no one. Every piece of fiction I have written fell into place by coincidence and intuition. Finding the perfect item for the main character to carry to complete the character arc at a thrift store in a small town I hadn't intended to visit. Having a dream that unmistakably tells me what the next direction in the story is. Running into an old friend who just happened to relay a story that sews up a gap in the plot.

Others may say this is simple observation. We don't know the half of what our brains are capable of. I agree. But I'm not very linear or logical by nature. I don't claim to know who or what god/dess is, but I know something else is a part of every living thing. I know that we are greater than the sum of our parts.

John Gardner's concept of entering a "fictive dream" applied to readers as well. He knew that a reader needed to be pulled irresistibly into a story or else there would be no reader, and he believed it was the writer's job to create that world. I believe the writer must also enter the fictive dream, not with the idea of manipulating it to her own ends, but with the presence to stop, stay awhile, and observe and record what happens there. An odd component of surrendering to this fictive dream is that it becomes as real, if not more real, than going to the grocery store, paying the bills, cleaning the toilets. We begin not only to understand the particular mythology of that dream, but to become a part of it. We form relationships of surprising depths with the inhabitants of that dream. We learn from them, and as we listen to and record what they have to say, we work through our own sorrows; we let go of what we didn't even know we were carrying, and we find ourselves, at the end of the writing process, a different person than the one who began the journey.

Jewell Parker Rhodes, author of the Marie Laveau novels, says that when we finish a novel, we should be changed. When I first began working seriously as a novelist, I thought she meant I would be older, maybe thinner. I had no idea that the change would be cellular, and that for a writer of fiction, our stories are our lifelong companions. They pull us; we don't pull them, into the next phase of our lives. Writer's block doesn't come from having nothing to say. It comes from being afraid to take the next step with our characters, so we create a frozen limbo to hold us up. This gives us the blessed opportunity to talk about writing rather than write. Many a writer has crashed his ship upon these tempting rocks.

But it is not a block. It is an unwillingness to surrender to the story.

As we breathe more deeply into the fictive dream, resistance loosens and we find ourselves in a place of deep surrender to our characters. It is here where relationships begin to form. Like the invisible playmates we had as children, the writer has the gift of continued communication with things unseen. A novel, by its sheer weight and breadth, is a formidable companion. It seeps into every aspect of our lives. We consult it before traveling. We think about the characters when we should be thinking about our students or our children or the speed of the car in front of us. They are always with us, and since a novel is, at best, a year commitment, most likely longer, we find ourselves in longer-term relationships with our characters than with some of our friends. When all else is bleak, the characters wrap their arms around us and give us shelter.

But it is the next piece of the relationship that sets me firmly in the "we are vessels" camp. The ending. Though I didn't think so at the time, I have come to feel gratitude for some of the early losses I've experienced. I learned that there is always another side to grief, and I have learned that with every ending comes a new beginning, as trite as that sounds when you're in the grip of sadness. But even knowing this, I was unprepared for what happened when I finished my first novel.

I don't know what I expected. Maybe the "Hallelujah Chorus" or a phone call from Bill Clinton, but I did not expect the silence. The bone dead silence of the room. I knew if I spoke, if I could think of anything to say, I would hear only my voice echoing from the bookshelves that surround my desk. I was alone, in a way that I had never been when my father died, or my lovers left, or we moved from my childhood home. As mysteriously as the characters had come to me, through dreams, newspaper clippings, jewelry pieces, they left. They simply left. If I had been in control of things, I would not have let that happen. Not then. Not so soon. Who knew in what other ways I would need them? But my agenda was not theirs and I was left with the awareness that I had been with them for a time and that time was over. I was powerless to do anything about it.

And I was unprepared.

I should have been . . . what? Happy? Relieved? Sad? I think I could have used any of those words to fill in the blank but the one I had to work with was: empty.

I was empty.

The first time it happened, I didn't know why. I went out with a friend to celebrate and ended up picking a terrible fight. I couldn't socialize. I felt raw, like my skin had been peeled back, leaving only quivering veins and tendons. I left my friend and walked down the street to where some horses were boarded. I touched the velvet noses, smelled the manure, and I wanted more than anything to become the horse. Eat. Drink. Run. Sleep. I felt I could handle that.

The next week was amplified and blurred. I was slow to make decisions. I could not communicate with people. I drove out to the desert, climbed a rock, and sat for five hours. It was all I could do. It never occurred to me that I was grieving.

"It's hard when they go," my former teacher said. "It is losing a part of yourself."

My sheets itched. The radio was too loud. My food was tasteless. I couldn't remember why I entered a room.

Grief.

Do you tell people you're grieving because your characters went away? Do you tell them you had no idea they would go away? That you thought they were yours and that you could dismiss them on your schedule? Will there be others? Will the next book be the same? What do you say to people who only inhabit one world, not two?

Nothing. You send a few e-mails to your writer friends and they respond. *Yes. Yes. That is how it is.* This comforts you, but only a little. You wonder if you are crazy and then remember that if you were crazy you wouldn't wonder whether you were or not; you would believe you were sane. You call former teachers.

I am without an immune system.

I am without definition.

I am without.

And the question that is underneath all the other questions.

What if no one comes again?

Teachers have no answers. Colleagues have no answers. It is the question underneath all their questions too. We don't know why the characters come, so we don't know if they will return.

"It is a leap of faith," my friend says. "We start a sentence and we have to trust that they will come and finish it. It is what we do."

If they don't go, there is no room for more to come.

When I finished my second novel, I was prepared for the leaving. It didn't soften the blow, but it did soften the surprise. We don't create our characters from clay and then build lives and deaths for them. They move into us and give us the words to tell their stories. They leave when the storytelling is done. We are left to pick up the pieces of our lives without them and start again, building new relationships with new unseen lives. Their departure is a signal that it is time to tell a different story.

I am certain the grieving can be explained by neurological factors and nice solid cognitive sciences, rather than my explanation of voices moving in and out of me like wind. But I do not find joy in a rational reason, and a rational reason will not sink into the nights I lay in bed and talked to my characters, argued with them, cried for them. A rational reason will not explain the things I have learned from them about my own life. The fictive dream is no less real to me than my flesh and blood life, and *this* life, *this* dream, is far too short to surrender what precious magic we are given to play with while a part of it.

Because deep writing requires us to form deep relationships with our characters and stories, we will naturally experience a time of solitude, sometimes loneliness, when we move from one project to the next. Know that this is normal. You are normal. You have done good work and you will do good work again.

Inhale. Exhale. Smile.

Touchstones

1. What is your relationship to solitude? What does it mean to you? How do you spend time alone? What distractions do you use to pull yourself away from solitude?

2. Write a monologue from the point of view of a character who has lived alone, away from community, since childhood. What does he or she have to say?

3. Choose a character you are currently having difficulty with and write a monologue from his or her point of view examining his or her views on loss and change. Write the story of the last time this character grieved.

4. Write a monologue from the point of view of a tree or animal examining the concept of solitude.

5. What comes up for you when you approach the end of a project? Do you resist the end? Do you skip ahead and try

to control it? Write about the "ending" process of a recent project.

6. Write a gratitude letter to the characters who have visited you in the past.

7. Create a ritual to mark the ending of a project. There are no rules here. Find the elements, the time, and the place that is meaningful for you.

27

STILLNESS

Just as one throws away old clothes and takes new ones, so, too, the soul, i.e., the dweller in the body, leaves old bodies and enters into new ones.

BHAGAVAD GITA 2:29

AT LAST. A RESTING PLACE. A place of true surrender. As with all the things I've been discussing, the source of this stillness is within you. Stillness is not "out there" in an isolated canyon. You can find stillness in the midst of a traffic jam or an argument with a friend. One of my yoga teachers says as we approach this place of stillness at the end of the practice, "The world can turn without your help for just a moment." This sentence can be helpful for letting go of responsibilities and belief systems about our ability to control things. Let your thoughts fall away like leaves. Let your body release its tension.

Before I talk about this point in the writing process, I'd like, if you're willing, for you to try something with your body. If you can, lie flat on the floor. If you have lower back trouble, you can put a blanket or pillow underneath your knees. Let your arms rest at your sides, palms up. Let your feet fall open. Begin to focus on your breath. Breathe in while counting to three, pause, then release with a sound, "Aaaahhhh." It's OK; no one is watching you. Do this two more times and then let your breathing return to normal. Begin to imagine your body as hollow, like a reed. It's a tunnel for the wave of your breath. Everything falls away but the breath. Sink deeper toward the earth. Your shoulders release their burdens. Your fingers are motionless and heavy. You are supported, held, by the floor and the earth beneath it. You are only breath. You follow that wave of breath in and out. No holding. No resisting. No trying to do anything. Lie like this for ten minutes before slowly bringing movement back to your fingers and toes. When you feel ready, roll onto your right side. Breathe. In your own time, slowly sit up. As you're ready, pick up your pen and write. Don't say anything, don't leave the room you're in, re-main as closely connected to the stillness as you can. Stop writing when you are done. Notice the stillness in the body and mind, no intentions, no desires. As each thought surfaces, release it without attachment.

This same place of stillness is present in the writing process too, if you allow for it. Our tendency is to run away from it, if we are even consciously aware that it's there. Think of this still place as the *kumbhaka,* the "in-between space" of your writing process. It is the place in between the breathing, the place in between the consciously doing and consciously not doing. It is empty, vast, and expansive. It is the pause in between that will allow you to make a bridge to the next project or idea. It gives you space to release what you've done and prepare for what is to come.

As you may have noticed, humans like to fill up empty spaces. We like to start right away on something new or chan-nel our energy right away into the next more exciting thing. The silence of the stillness can scare us. Stay here awhile. This is the space in between, the web reaching from one wall to the next. Don't worry. You won't get stuck. You'll have to inhale again, but by lingering in this place you honor what you've done. You clear out any residual droppings from that project. You cleanse your being, and in doing so, you're preparing the way for unexpected delights. There's no secret code, no special key, no single magic phrase I can give you to demystify this writer's journey. What I can give you is ancient wisdom: When you write, write. When you play, play. When you love, love. Experience each part of your path fully, and as you step from one stage into the next, release the previous stage completely so you can continue to always step fully into each present moment. This is life. It's not better over there, or with the newest computer program, or with a more ergonomic chair.

This is life, right here, right now. Don't lose sight of that by desiring the future or longing for the past. This is it, all of it, and it is full and complete. From this space, this place of perfection, bring the world your stories. From this union of body, mind, and spirit, write.

EPILOGUE

You might enjoy using this epilogue as a reminder of the key components of the writing process. Perhaps you could post it on your computer or above your writing table. May it help you maintain focus, awareness, and compassion for yourself and your journey.

Write.
Build your foundation by reading, writing,
    engaging with other writers, and revising.
Write.
Stretch yourself. Submit your work. When it
    comes back, look at it again. See what you can
    do to make it better, stronger, more precise
    and aligned. Send it out again. When it comes
    back, look at it again. Continue on.
Write.
Return often to your foundation. It's easy to lose
    sight of the basics if you are reaching too far
    forward. You'll topple over without grounding
    yourself.
Write.
Stretch. Collapse. Stretch. Collapse. Stretch.
    Remain steady.
Write.

Move deeper into your foundation work. Practice
dialogue only for a week. Practice plotting or
characterization. Stay focused on a single craft
aspect. Watch it open up for you into volumes
you'd never anticipated. With humility, laugh,
and begin again.

May you find balance within yourself and with the world
around you, and may every act sow seeds of peace, connection, and community.

RECOMMENDED RESOURCES

This is certainly not a complete list of all the great resources available to you on this journey of writing and self-exploration. I've compiled what I think are solid foundational books in the various genres and the two primary writing stages, as well as a book on publishing your work. I've also included reference books on yoga and Zen practices. Any of these books will provide you a starting place to begin your own exploration.

Addonizio, Kim, and Dorianne Laux. *The Poet's Companion: A Guide to the Pleasures of Writing Poetry.* New York: W. W. Norton and Co., 1997. Textbook on contemporary poetry, complete with many wonderful writing exercises. Prewriting and revision stages.

Brandeis, Gayle. *Fruitflesh.* New York: HarperCollins, 2002. Sensuous writing exercises based in the body. Prewriting stage.

Burroway, Janet, and Elizabeth Stuckey-French. *Writing Fiction.* 7th ed. New York: Pearson Longman, 2006. The most comprehensive text I've found on the craft of fiction. Every chapter is packed with pertinent craft information. Prewriting and revision stages.

Cameron, Julia. *The Artist's Way: A Spiritual Path to Higher Creativity.* New York: Putnam, 2002. Great guide for kick-starting your creativity. Prewriting stage.

Campbell, Joseph. *The Hero with a Thousand Faces.* Princeton, N. J.: Princeton University Press, reprint edition, 1972. Seminal work of comparative mythologist, Joseph Campbell. Discusses the hero's journey, the monomyth, and the roles of myths in cultures around the world. Highly recommended for anyone wanting to write stories.

Chiarella, Tom. *Writing Dialogue: How to Create Memorable Voices and Fictional Conversations That Crackle with Wit, Tension, and Nuance.* Cincinnati: Story Press, 1998. Funny, accessible book that blows open the mysteries of literary dialogue. Prewriting and revision stages.

Chödrön, Pema. *The Places That Scare You: A Guide to Fearlessness in Difficult Times.* Boston: Shambhala Publications, 2001. Guidance from a Buddhist perspective on tackling the dark places within.

Desai, Yogi Amrit. *Amrit Yoga and the Yoga Sutras: Amrit Yoga and Its Roots in Patanjali's Ashtanga Yoga.* Sumneytown, Penn: Yoga Network International, 2002. Guide from the founder of Amrit yoga on the ancient yoga teachings.

Dogen. *Beyond Thinking: A Guide to Zen Meditation.* Boston: Shambhala Publications, 2004. Practical teachings from one of Japan's greatest Zen masters.

Feuerstein, Georg. *The Yoga Tradition: Its History, Philosophy, Literature and Practice.* Prescott, Ariz.: Hohm Press, 2001. A good accessible overview of the yoga tradition.

Gardner, John. *The Art of Fiction: Notes on Craft for Young Writers.* New York: Vintage Books, 1991. A classic. Gardner presents a no-frills approach to fiction writing. He plays hardball. Prewriting and revision stages.

———. *On Becoming a Novelist.* New York: W. W. Norton and Company, 1999. A text focusing on what it takes, psychologically, to be a novelist. Fascinating reading for anyone hoping to write novels. Prewriting and revision stages.

Goldberg, Natalie. *Writing Down the Bones: Freeing the Writer Within.* Boston: Shambhala Publications, 2006. An inspiring international classic focusing on prewriting.

Gordon, Karen Elizabeth. *The Deluxe Transitive Vampire: A Handbook of Grammar for the Innocent, the Eager, and the Doomed.* New York: Pantheon, 1993. For the grammatically challenged writer. You too can learn the complexities of grammar. Revision stage.

————. *The New Well-Tempered Sentence: A Punctuation Handbook for the Innocent, the Eager, and the Doomed.* New York: Houghton Mifflin, 1993. Sentence level grammatical insights. No advanced grammar concepts. Revision stage.

Hanh, Thich Nhat. *Peace Is Every Step: The Path of Mindfulness in Everyday Life.* New York: Bantam, 1992. Gentle guidance in mindfulness and loving-kindness.

Herman, Jeff. *Write the Perfect Book Proposal: Ten That Sold and Why.* 2nd ed. New York: Wiley, 2001. Useful, practical book on writing book proposals to acquire an agent or publisher. Revision stage.

Iyengar, B.K.S. *Light on Yoga.* New York: Schocken, 1995. In depth study of the yogic path.

Jung, Carl. *Memories, Dreams, Reflections.* New York: Vintage, 1989. Essentially a memoir, Jung explores his uncovering of his unconscious in an accessible, valuable way.

King, Stephen. *On Writing.* New York: Pocket, 2002. Nuts and bolts guidance from one of America's most prolific writers. King plays hardball, too. Prewriting and revision stages.

Kowit, Steve. *In the Palm of Your Hand: The Poet's Portable Workshop.* Gardiner, Me.: Tillbury House Publishers, 1995. Another excellent poetry text, complete with many exercises. Prewriting and revision stages.

Lamott, Anne. *Bird by Bird: Some Instructions on Writing and Life.* New York: Anchor, 1995. A classic, easy-to-read account of the writer's life. Prewriting stage.

Lee, John. *Writing from the Body: For Writers, Artists, and Dreamers Who Long to Free Their Voices.* New York: St. Martin's Griffin, 1994.

Wonderful body-based exercises for writers of all genres. Prewriting stage.

Levitt, Peter. *Fingerpainting on the Moon: Writing and Creativity as a Path to Freedom.* New York: Harmony, 2003. Beautifully written, gentle guide to the inner landscape of your writing. Prewriting stage.

Maharshi, Sri Ramana. *Be as You Are: The Teachings of Sri Ramana Maharshi.* Edited by David Godman. New Delhi, India: Penguin Books, 1992. Unexplainable. Read it for yourself and notice what you feel.

Rosen, Richard. *The Yoga of Breath: A Step-by-Step Guide to Pranayama.* Boston: Shambhala Publications, 2002. Comprehensive and accessible step-by-step guide to pranayama.

Rumi, Jalal al-Din. *Essential Rumi.* Translated by Coleman Barks. New York: HarperCollins, 1995. Mystical lyric poetry and prose.

Simmons, Jerry. *Inside the Business of Publishing: What Writers Need to Know.* Scottsdale, Ariz., 2005. A self-published book available on the author's website: www.writersreaders.com. Comprehensive guide to the world of publishing. Extremely valuable when you reach the point of contacting agents. Revision stage.

Strunk, William Jr., and E.B. White. *Elements of Style.* 4th ed. New York: Longman, 2000. The definitive style guide. Buy it. Read it. Know it. Revision stage.

Suzuki, Shunryu. *Zen Mind, Beginner's Mind.* Boston: Weatherhill, 1973. Perhaps the most-read book in the West on Zen teaching. It's a great companion book on the writer's path. Prewriting and revision stages.

Vogler, Christopher. *The Writer's Journey: Mythic Structure for Writers.* 2nd ed. Studio City, Calif.: Michael Wiese Productions, 1998. A very useful guide for structuring and plotting based on Joseph Campbell's hero's journey. Excellent for revision stage.

Watts, Alan. *The Way of Zen.* New York: Vintage, 1999. For those who would like more information on Zen teaching and philosophy.

Whyte, David. *Clear Mind, Wild Heart.* Audio CD. Louisville, Col.: Sounds True, 2002. A poet's interpretation of the writing and living process. A delight. Prewriting stage.

Zinsser, William. *Inventing the Truth: The Art and Craft of Memoir.* New York: Mariner Books, 1998. Essays on the craft of memoir from prominent memoirists. Prewriting and revision stages.

————. *On Writing Well: The Classic Guide to Writing Nonfiction.* 30th anniversary ed. New York: HarperCollins, 2006. Just like it sounds. The classic on the craft of nonfiction writing. Prewriting and revision stages.

Zweig, Connie, and Jeremiah Abrams. *Meeting the Shadow: The Hidden Power of the Dark Side of Human Nature.* New York: Tarcher, 1991. A wonderful assortment of essays dealing with the shadow side of the human psyche. Accessible to the lay person.

ABOUT THE AUTHOR

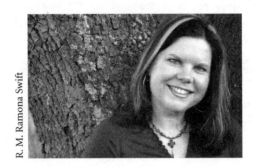

R. M. Ramona Swift

LARAINE HERRING holds an MFA in creative writing and an MA in counseling psychology. She has developed numerous workshops that use writing as a tool for healing grief and loss. She is the author of *Lost Fathers: How Women Heal from Adolescent Father Loss,* and *Monsoons,* a book of short stories. Her short stories, poems, and essays have appeared in national and local publications. Her fiction has won the Barbara Deming Award for Women and her nonfiction work has been nominated for a Pushcart Prize. She currently teaches creative writing in Prescott, Arizona. Learn more about Laraine at www.laraineherring.com.